Healing
HEARTBURN

A JOHNS HOPKINS

PRESS HEALTH BOOK

Healing

HEARTBURN

LAWRENCE J. CHESKIN, M.D.

BRIAN E. LACY, M.D., Ph.D.

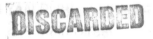

THE JOHNS HOPKINS UNIVERSITY PRESS
Baltimore & London

Note to the Reader: *This book is not meant to substitute for the medical care of persons with gastroesophageal reflux disease or other medical problems, and treatment should not be based solely on its contents. Instead, treatment must be developed in a dialogue between an individual and his or her physician. Our book has been written to help with that dialogue.*

The names in the case studies presented in this book are fictitious.

© 2002 The Johns Hopkins University Press
All rights reserved. Published 2002
Printed in the United States of America on acid-free paper
9 8 7 6 5 4 3 2 1

The Johns Hopkins University Press
2715 North Charles Street
Baltimore, Maryland 21218-4363
www.press.jhu.edu

Black-and-white illustrations by Jacqueline Schaffer.

Library of Congress Cataloging-in-Publication Data
Cheskin, Lawrence J.
Healing heartburn / Lawrence J. Cheskin, Brian E. Lacy.
   p. cm.
Includes bibliographical references and index.
ISBN 0-8018-6868-8 (hardback)—ISBN 0-8018-6869-6 (paperback)

1. Heartburn—Popular works. I. Lacy, Brian E. II. Title.
RC815.7 .C48 2002
616.3'32—dc21

2001002426

A catalog record for this book is available from the British Library.

*This book is dedicated to the memory of Patrick Lacy.
As a father, he was patient, kind, generous, and encouraging.
In both his personal and professional endeavors, he treated
everyone he encountered, regardless of their position or
achievements, with respect and kindness, and, in doing so,
inspired those around him to do the same.*

Contents

Preface   ix

Acknowledgments   xiii

Part I   INTRODUCTION

Chapter 1   What Is Gastroesophageal Reflux Disease?   3

Chapter 2   What Goes Wrong in GERD, and Where It Goes Wrong   11

Part II   SYMPTOMS *&* DIAGNOSIS

Chapter 3   What Are the Symptoms of GERD?   27

Chapter 4   Diagnosing GERD   47

Part III   TREATMENT: THE FOUR-STEP APPROACH

Chapter 5   Step 1: Lifestyle Modifications   69

Chapter 6   Step 2: Over-the-Counter Medicines   80

Chapter 7   Steps 3 & 4: Prescription Medicines and
            Surgery   96

Part IV   COMPLICATIONS & SPECIAL SITUATIONS

Chapter 8   Complications of GERD   115

Chapter 9   GERD in Children, Pregnant Women, the Older Patient,
            and the Bed-Bound   135

Part V   THE FUTURE

Chapter 10 A Look into the Future: Diagnosing and Treating GERD
            and Complications of GERD   153

            Abbreviations   171

            Glossary   173

            Where to Go for Further Information & Support   181

            Index   183

Preface

Nearly everyone has at one time or another experienced heartburn, the sensation of burning discomfort or pain behind the breastbone that is often brought on by eating a large meal. In fact, heartburn is the most common gastrointestinal disorder in the United States: more than 4 in 10 adult Americans suffer from heartburn each month. Although the word *heartburn* is commonly used to describe both the burning feeling and the disorder that is causing the burning feeling, heartburn is really just one symptom of the disorder that is more properly known as *gastroesophageal reflux disease,* or *GERD*. This term more accurately describes the cause of heartburn, which is the *reflux* (or backing up) of acid from the stomach *(gastrum)* into the esophagus. In this book we will use the terms *heartburn* and *gastroesophageal reflux disease* more or less interchangeably, because *heartburn* is the term most people recognize.

We have written this book with several goals in mind:

* to help educate you about GERD
* to overcome (or eliminate) misconceptions about this disease
* to help you recognize both common and uncommon symptoms of GERD

* to describe available treatments, both medical and surgical
* to allow you to take charge of your life by dealing with this common problem

When someone visits a physician because of heartburn or other symptoms of gastroesophageal reflux disease, the physician will generally approach the problem with four major goals in mind. The first is to correctly identify the problem. This task may be relatively straightforward, based on the patient's history and symptoms, for example. Or it may require one or more trials of medications as well as diagnostic tests. Once a diagnosis has been made, the physician focuses on his or her second goal, which is to determine the best treatment plan for this patient, a treatment plan that will eliminate symptoms, make the patient feel better, and treat the underlying disease. The physician's third goal is to educate the patient about the nature of the problem and the treatment plan. Patients who are well informed about their medical conditions and the importance of treatment are often better able to monitor their symptoms and identify minor problems before they become serious. Finally, the physician will work with the patient to prevent any potential complications of the disease and, if necessary, to treat complications that develop despite the best efforts to prevent them.

As physicians ourselves, we strongly believe that an essential part of every physician's job in providing the best treatment is to inform and educate the patient, as much as possible, about the nature of his or her illness. This knowledge helps people deal with illness because they understand why they suffer from a particular health condition, and helps them prevent or minimize future problems. When people understand their bodies and their diseases and disorders, they and their physicians can make the most out of every visit, because they can meaningfully discuss the course of the disease and all of the treatment options. In this way the patient and physician work together as a team to form a treatment plan. There is another advantage to knowledge, as well: patients who understand their own bodies are better able to make rational lifestyle and dietary choices that can prevent GERD from occurring and recurring.

This book is divided into five parts. In Part I, two chapters explain who gets GERD and why, as well as what parts of the anatomy are involved and how they can cause trouble.

Part II focuses on symptoms and diagnosis. In this part of the book, Chapter 3 provides an "up close and personal" description of heartburn as well as other possible symptoms of GERD, including regurgitation, wheezing, cough, and hoarseness. Chapter 4 explains what's involved in the diagnostic tests used to evaluate people who are suspected of having GERD.

Chapter 5 begins Part III, the treatment section of the book, with a discussion of lifestyle factors that can be changed to help reduce the risk of suffering from GERD symptoms. Chapters 6 and 7 are all about medications, both over-the-counter and prescription, and Chapter 7 also describes the surgery that is occasionally necessary in the treatment of GERD.

In Part IV, Chapter 8 provides detailed information on the complications of GERD along with information on how these complications are treated. Chapter 9 takes a slightly different view of GERD, looking at how the disease affects special populations, such as children and pregnant women.

Part V concludes the book with a single chapter that looks at promising new ways to diagnose and treat GERD. At the back of the book the reader will find a list of abbreviations used in this book, a glossary of terms and their definitions, and a list of places to go for additional information and support.

We hope you find this book to be informative and useful. We hope it answers all of your questions about heartburn and allows you to take charge of this problem.

To your good health!

Acknowledgments

Writing a book requires the combined efforts of many people who work tirelessly behind the scenes, often without credit. To counteract that tendency, we would like to thank our editor at the Johns Hopkins University Press, Jacqueline Wehmueller. This book would still be in the planning stages if not for her. We also owe thanks to Mary Yates, our copy editor, who did a tremendous job blending different writing styles and pulling the book together.

We are very grateful for the opportunity to work with our many patients who suffer from heartburn. We hope that we have been able to alleviate their symptoms and improve their quality of life.

We thank our families for their unwavering support during the writing process. We hope to make it up to them in the future for their many sacrifices while we wrote this book.

Part I

INTRODUCTION

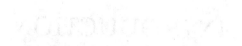

Chapter 1

What Is Gastroesophageal Reflux Disease?

"It's just heartburn." Many people ignore the symptoms of gastroesophageal reflux disease (GERD), or else treat themselves routinely with Tums or Rolaids, without understanding that it *isn't* "just heartburn." While heartburn is a common symptom and GERD is a common disorder, it still hurts, and it can be dangerous. Let's look at a fairly typical case.

Joe is a 43-year-old sales manager who had always thought of himself as healthy. But he got a scare one night last September, after closing an important deal with clients at a fine steakhouse in town. Joe ordered prime rib—only the "queen-sized" portion, as he had been watching his weight—and a Caesar salad. He shared a bottle of red wine with his clients, and he topped off the meal with a piece of Black Forest cake and a cup of black coffee. On his way out of the restaurant he popped a couple of peppermints into his mouth.

After dropping his clients off at their hotel, Joe—feeling pleasantly stuffed but not uncomfortable—headed to his house in the suburbs, 40 minutes away. Close to home he started to feel queasy, so he loosened his belt. It felt good finally to get home and put on a loose-fitting robe and talk over the day with his wife, Marie.

Lying down in bed to watch the 10 o'clock news with a diet soda, Joe felt a bit warm, but after he sat up and belched, he felt better. It had been a long day, and he could barely keep his eyes open during the news. He got up, brushed his teeth, and went back to bed to sleep.

Tired as he was, Joe just couldn't get comfortable. He rolled from his back to his side to his stomach and back again. Gradually he noticed an uncomfortable sensation down low in his chest—a heavy, hot sensation deep inside, behind the breastbone. He shifted again in bed, but now he was even more uncomfortable. The sensation was moving up inside his chest toward his neck and throat. Joe was scared, and he sat up in bed quickly as a wave of nausea hit him. He staggered to the bathroom, uncertain what to do once he got there. The nausea passed, but he tasted something sour in the back of his throat. And the feeling in his chest was still there. It was a burning sensation now. For the first time Joe wondered if he could be having a heart attack.

He rinsed his month out with cold water, then drank some water. That seemed to help, and he went back to bed. The burning was still there, however, and he tossed and turned some more. Marie woke up and asked him what was wrong.

"I don't know. It feels like my chest is on fire, but I didn't even eat anything spicy."

"Sounds like heartburn," Marie told him. "You've had that before."

"You think that's all it is? It's silly to even say this, but for a minute there I thought I was having a heart attack."

"Try some of my antacids. There's a bottle on the top shelf of the medicine cabinet. If they don't work, maybe we should go to the emergency room."

Joe went back to the bathroom, found the bottle, and read the label: "For temporary relief of heartburn and other stomach ailments. Take 1 tablespoon every 2 to 3 hours as needed."

"Real men don't need a tablespoon to measure medicine," he thought, and took a big slug straight from the bottle. The stuff tasted pretty bad, kind of chalky, but tolerable. He rinsed his month out afterward, then took another, smaller, swallow for good measure, feeling a little less certain about the size of his first swallow, and rinsed his mouth again.

Remarkably, within a minute or two Joe began to feel better. The burning fire became a dull ache and then went away entirely. Joe went back to bed and slept until the morning alarm greeted him with tales of traffic jams. A new day had begun, and he quickly forgot about the unpleasant experience of the previous night.

But Joe's symptoms returned the next weekend, after a cookout. This time he knew what to expect and headed straight for the medicine cabinet. He was amazed at how quickly he felt better once he drank the antacid. Antacid. *Antiacid*. How about that! Maybe he should stop drinking orange juice—that was acid, wasn't it? And maybe he shouldn't eat such big meals before going to bed. He'd try to cut that out.

Once or twice a week for the next several months Joe felt twinges of heartburn. He was becoming an expert on the different flavors of liquid antacid, and he carried chewable antacid tablets with him in his car. Although they tasted better than the liquids, the tablets didn't work as well. "Typical," he complained to Marie. "If it tastes bad, it works better."

One night Joe had a particularly bad bout of heartburn that didn't go away for several hours, even though he took dose after dose of liquid antacid. He asked around the next day at work and found out that a lot of other people had heartburn, too. One of his fellow sufferers recommended the newer antacids that come in pill form: Pepcid AC or Zantac or Tagamet.

Joe started taking Zantac regularly, along with liquid or tablet antacids when he needed them. This routine worked better, and he'd go for a couple of weeks without having much heartburn. Twice he stopped taking the pills when it seemed that the symptoms were gone, only to be rudely reminded a day or two later that he still had the problem. Then, after another couple of painful episodes, he decided to see his family doctor about the problem. It had been 10 months since his first attack.

After listening to Joe's stories and examining him, Dr. Alfred Johnson, an internist, was fairly certain that Joe had heartburn and nothing more, such as an ulcer. Dr. Johnson started Joe on a stronger, prescription-strength, antacid medicine, one of the class of drugs called *histamine type 2 blockers*, or H_2-*blockers* for short. This type of medication blocks the action of *histamine*, a potent stimulator of acid release in the stomach.

Is Joe's story unusual? No. In fact, the statistics are remarkable. In the United States, more than 40 percent of adults surveyed by telephone report experiencing symptoms of heartburn at least as often as once a month. This is more than 60 million people! Further, at least 7 percent of adult Americans report having symptoms every day. Thirteen percent of adults use over-the-counter antacids (also known as *anti-acids*) at least twice a week. Joe has a fairly severe case of GERD and needs prescription medications to control his symptoms, and this is not uncommon, either.

The medical name for what all these people are suffering from is *gastroesophageal reflux disease,* or *GERD.* GERD is a medical condition in which stomach acid comes into contact with the esophagus (the swallowing tube connecting the back of the mouth and the stomach) and produces any number of symptoms, such as:

* heartburn, which is usually perceived as a hot, burning, dull ache or pain behind the breastbone
* acid regurgitation, which is the sensation that acid has found its way all the way up from the stomach into the mouth, causing a sour taste in the mouth
* excessive belching (which requires no explanation)
* water brash, which is the sudden appearance of a large amount of saliva in the mouth
* difficulty swallowing or painful swallowing

As we saw with Joe, the symptoms of GERD can be unpleasant, painful, and even frightening. Often they are life-disrupting. And, as we'll see when Joe's story continues below, GERD can cause complications that are more serious, including esophagitis, esophageal strictures, and the condition called *Barrett's esophagus* (discussed in Chapter 8). While GERD is usually no more than a medical annoyance, in the case of someone with the complication of Barrett's esophagus it is a risk for cancer of the esophagus. Not only are GERD-related complications common, they may occur even when the person has mild—or even no—heartburn symptoms.

The prescription Dr. Johnson wrote for Joe was for ranitidine hydrochloride (Zantac), 300 mg po q 6PM. This translates into one pill of 300-milligram strength by mouth (*p.o.* means *per os,* which is Latin for "by mouth") every evening at six. (The 300-mg strength is four times as much medicine as the nonprescription strength, of 75 mg.) Joe was told not to skip medicines on days when he had no symptoms. Dr. Johnson emphasized that Joe needed to take the medication every day for a while—and perhaps for the rest of his life—to control his symptoms and prevent them from returning.

Joe did as he was told, at least for a few weeks, and got complete relief from his heartburn. When the prescription ran out, he called for a refill and told Dr. Johnson how well the prescription-strength medicine was working.

Unfortunately, the relief was temporary, but that's because over time Joe began to take the medicine less faithfully. His heartburn got worse, and when the last refill of his prescription ran out, Joe began taking nonprescription medicines again. He took them, contrary to the label directions, two or three at a time, hoping to achieve the dose of his prescription pills. But not only was this ineffective (and possibly dangerous), it also cost more than the prescription pills. Joe returned to Dr. Johnson, who reexamined him, found no change or alarming new symptoms, and put him on an even stronger medicine, omeprazole (Prilosec). This was the most powerful anti-acid medicine available at the time, in the class of medications called *proton-pump inhibitors.*

Relief! Just like the old days, when liquid antacids had been enough. Joe felt better, but he was worried. Why was it getting harder and harder to control his heartburn? A few months later, after he started to skip or miss doses of his medication, Joe's symptoms returned with a vengeance and caught up with him earlier and earlier in the day. He and his wife were seriously concerned. Dr. Johnson decided to refer Joe to a *gastroenterologist* (a specialist in diseases of the gastrointestinal tract) for further evaluation.

The gastroenterologist, Dr. Andrea Martines, went over Joe's history, performed a physical examination (including a rectal exam to check for blood in the stool, among other things), ordered some simple blood tests, and carefully reviewed the information about Joe's medical history that Dr. Johnson had sent over to her.

She agreed that, most likely, Joe's problem was indeed a severe case of GERD and that acid refluxing (moving upward) from the stomach into the esophagus was causing it. She explained to Joe that it was best, in someone of his age, for a doctor to take a look into his esophagus and stomach to see if there was any visible damage and to determine whether another condition, such as an ulcer, was responsible for Joe's symptoms.

Joe was scheduled later that same week for a diagnostic procedure called an *upper endoscopy,* also known as *esophagogastroduodenoscopy,* or *EGD* for short. (The letters denote the three regions of the upper gastrointestinal tract that can be seen using this technique: the *esophagus,* the *gastrum* [Latin for *stomach*], and the *duodenum* [the upper small intestine].) The only thing Joe needed to do to prepare for this procedure was to not eat or drink anything for eight hours before the EGD. Dr. Martines might also have performed a 24-hour pH test, another test for GERD, if Joe's diagnosis was still in doubt after the EGD. (Both the EGD and the 24-hour pH test are described in Chapter 4.)

The EGD evidence indicated that Joe did have GERD. In fact, he also had a complication of GERD called *esophagitis.* Esophagitis is a condition most commonly caused by acid reflux. The esophagus can become inflamed and irritated by harsh stomach acid when someone has had uncontrolled acid reflux disease for some time. Evidence of esophagitis can be easily seen through the lighted fiberoptic tube called the *endoscope* that is threaded down the esophagus to perform this test. A photograph of the reddened, irritated lining of Joe's esophagus taken through the endoscope is shown in plate 2 (facing page 130). Joe did not have a stomach ulcer or a duodenal ulcer (an ulcer in the duodenum) or any sign of cancer. In addition to esophagitis, however, he did have a small *hiatal hernia,* a condition that is not a symptom or complication of GERD but is sometimes associated with GERD (see Chapter 2).

During the upper endoscopy, Dr. Martines took biopsies (samples of tissue) of Joe's esophagus. The biopsies were studied under a microscope by a pathologist, who was able to identify different causes and types of inflammation from the appearance of the tissues. Joe's irritated-looking esophagus, according to the pathologist who looked at his biopsies, was caused by acid reflux and did not show any evidence of cancer or the precancerous condition called *Barrett's esophagus* (see Chapter 8).

Dr. Martines prescribed double the dose of the proton-pump inhibitor that Joe was taking, to help ensure that his esophagus healed completely. This time Joe was convinced that he needed to take the medication faithfully, and he did so. His symptoms disappeared on this higher dose of medicine, and they have remained fully controlled ever since. The medication costs $1,800 each year, but Joe is fortunate, because his health insurance plan covers all but a small portion of this cost.

Joe's case history illustrates many of the common risk factors, symptoms, and treatments of GERD, and we will refer to Joe's story for the remainder of this chapter to illustrate what is known about who is at highest risk for GERD and what can be done to avoid or minimize the symptoms of it.

GERD affects men and women about equally. Although far fewer children than adults have GERD, GERD can be a cause of chronic vomiting in infancy and childhood, and it may affect a child's ability to grow normally. As we discuss in Chapter 9, pregnancy can cause or increase the symptoms of GERD; about one-quarter of all pregnant woman suffer from heartburn daily, and more than half of all pregnant women have less frequent heartburn.

GERD has affected a large proportion of people living in the United States and all Western countries for a very long time, but only in the past 20 years has it been called *GERD*. Before that it was simply called *heartburn*. *Heartburn* is now considered a poor term to use because it implies that the source of discomfort is the heart. While GERD-like symptoms occasionally turn out to be true cardiac pain *(angina pectoris)*, true GERD and its classic symptom of heartburn have nothing to do with the heart. (As we mentioned in the Preface, however, in this book we use both terms, *heartburn* and *gastroesophageal reflux disease*, because so many people are accustomed to the word *heartburn*.)

We use Joe's story to illustrate GERD for a number of reasons. First, his symptoms are typical of GERD. Second, those symptoms got worse despite treatment, and therefore Joe's care involved a number of the steps of progressively more intensive diagnosis and treatment that we normally recommend for persistent GERD. It is best to start out with simple lifestyle measures, such as a change in dietary habits, then add over-the-counter (OTC) medicines like antacids and OTC H_2-blockers, then move to prescription-strength H_2-blockers, and finally to proton-pump inhibitors if these earlier steps of treatment fail to control the symptoms adequately. (These steps are described in Part III of this book.) For most people, only the first step or two of treatment is needed.

Finally, we use Joe as an illustration because he has some characteristics and habits that put him in a high-risk category for developing GERD and its complications. Did you spot the relevant details in his story? They are:

* Joe likes rich, fatty foods such as steaks and sauces and desserts. These kinds of foods can decrease the pressure in the muscular ring, or sphincter, that controls the lower esophagus, and they can also slow the emptying of the stomach. Both of these situations can lead to heartburn symptoms.
* Joe is overweight, which increases the risk that acid will reflux (or come up) into his esophagus, causing heartburn.
* Joe is a drinking man. Like rich foods, alcohol also lowers the pressure in the lower esophageal sphincter and increases the risk of GERD.
* Joe makes the mistake of lying down soon after a large meal, which puts further strain on an already relaxed lower esophageal sphincter, promoting reflux of acid into the esophagus.

For people reading this book who do some of the same things Joe does, the bad news is that these lifestyle factors can cause GERD. The good news, on the other hand, is that by changing these and other lifestyle factors, many people can decrease the severity of their GERD symptoms or can avoid developing such symptoms altogether.

In this chapter we have provided a brief description of GERD and its symptoms and complications, and we have introduced a number of factors that can cause GERD. We have briefly described what's involved in making a diagnosis of GERD, and we have sketched out the four steps of treatment that are generally recommended to relieve the symptoms of GERD. In the rest of this book we will provide more detailed information on all of these issues: symptoms, diagnosis, treatment, and complications. First, though, let's turn, in Chapter 2, to the anatomy of the upper gastrointestinal tract and take a closer look at where in the body the problems of GERD come about. We'll also look again at some of the causes of GERD and describe the difference between a hiatal hernia and gastroesophageal reflux disease, because the two disorders are closely linked and often confused.

What Goes Wrong in GERD, and Where It Goes Wrong

To understand gastroesophageal reflux disease, you first need to understand the structure and function of the digestive tract. This chapter describes the digestive tract, particularly the stomach and esophagus, and explains how abnormalities or dysfunction of the stomach or the esophagus can produce GERD. We will also explain hiatal hernias and how they are related to GERD.

The Big Picture: From Food to Waste

Figure 2.1 illustrates the organs that compose the gastrointestinal tract, a muscular tube over 30 feet in length that extends from the mouth to the anus. As one might expect, the various organs have different functions. Nevertheless, all the organs work together to accomplish the dual purposes of the digestive system: first, to extract liquid and nourishment from the food we eat and, second, to eliminate the waste material that's left over once the liquid and nutrients have been extracted. Food travels from the mouth down the esophagus into the stomach, where much of the digestion (breaking the food down into very tiny bits) takes place. Once it leaves the stomach, the material travels

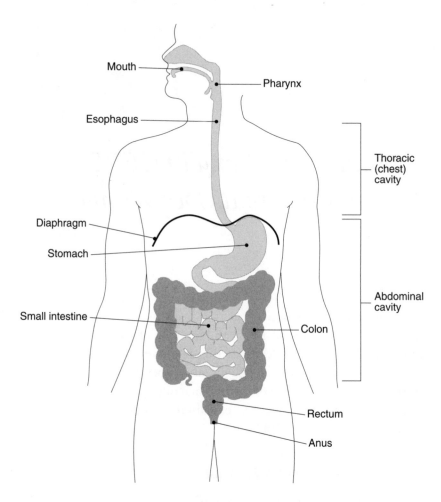

Figure 2.1. Overview of the gastrointestinal tract. Note how the esophagus resides in the thoracic (chest) cavity, while the stomach is located below the diaphragm, in the abdominal cavity.

through the small intestine and then through the large intestine (also called the *colon*) and rectum before exiting the body through the anus. Along the route, nutrients and liquid are absorbed by the body and carried by blood vessels to other parts of the body.

To propel the food from one part of the gastrointestinal tract to the next, muscles in the walls of the esophagus, stomach, and intestine contract and relax automatically and rhythmically (a process called *peristalsis*). The stomach mixes and grinds food and breaks it up into small particles that are then passed into the small intestine, the primary site for absorption of nutrients, vitamins, and minerals. Finally, the colon and rectum concentrate, store, and then eliminate waste products.

A Closer Look

As far as GERD is concerned, the two "trouble areas" of the gastrointestinal tract are the esophagus and the stomach. These two organs are directly connected, but they lie in different areas of the body. The esophagus resides in the thoracic (chest) cavity, the area above the diaphragm where the heart, the trachea (windpipe), and the lungs are also found. (The diaphragm is the dome-shaped layer of muscle and tendon that contracts and expands to pull air into and out of the lungs.) The stomach is located below the diaphragm, in the abdominal cavity (the abdomen). The abdominal cavity also contains the liver, intestines, spleen, kidneys, gallbladder, and pancreas. There are openings in the diaphragm that make it possible for major blood vessels and the organs of the digestive system to communicate between the chest and the abdomen. Such an opening is called a *hiatus*. The point where the esophagus passes through the diaphragm—through an opening called the *esophageal hiatus*—is a potential problem site. As we will discuss later, if this opening widens, it can create hiatal hernias as well as other types of hernias.

The Esophagus

The esophagus is a muscular tube approximately 10 inches long that begins in the throat and ends in the stomach (see Figure 2.1). The primary function of the esophagus is to propel food and liquid from the mouth into the stomach. The esophagus is connected to the mouth in an area at the back of the throat called the *pharynx*. The pharynx is essentially an open space located behind the nose and mouth. Liquids pass through the esophagus from the pharynx to the stomach in only one second. The trip for solid foods takes slightly longer—up to several seconds. The esophagus functions fairly automatically: once food is swallowed, it is propelled directly into the stomach by a series of muscular contractions that do not require any conscious thought. The muscles of the esophagus are very strong and can easily overcome even gravity. It is possible to eat and drink (carefully!) while standing on one's head.

The Stomach

Although most people point to their belly button when they refer to their stomach, most of the stomach is located up much higher: in many people it is as high as right underneath the ribs. The stomach is a hollow J-shaped muscular organ that lies beneath the diaphragm in the abdominal cavity (see Figure 2.2). The stomach functions in part as a temporary storage site for food, and its walls have the amazing ability to relax and expand to accommodate large amounts of food (up to two quarts), such as after a large holiday meal.

The main function of the stomach, however, is to mix and grind food and then propel it into the small intestine so that it can be further digested and absorbed. Food leaves the stomach through a muscular opening called the *pylorus,* but only after each piece of food has been ground up into tiny particles (usually less than one millimeter in size, about the size of the head of a pin).

The lining of the stomach contains millions of glands that produce various chemicals called *gastric secretions,* two of the most important of which are hydrochloric acid and pepsinogen. Hydrochloric acid breaks down food particles and sterilizes the food, and thus helps with the early stages of digestion. (This same acid, however, plays a major role in the development of GERD and peptic ulcers.) Pepsinogen is a type of substance that is known as an *enzyme precursor.* It is released from the stomach glands in an inactive form, and is then activated and converted into pepsin, its active form, by hydrochloric acid. Pepsin is a special type of enzyme that helps speed up the breakdown of proteins in foods or liquids. (Enzymes help catalyze a chemical reaction. That is, they help speed up or enhance the action of other chemicals.) As

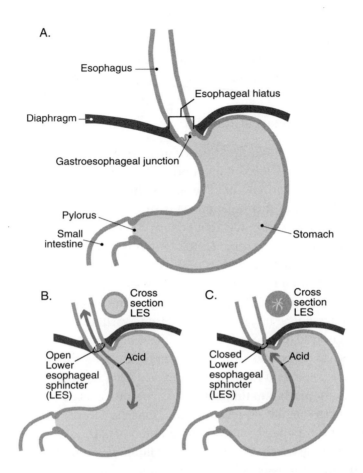

Figure 2.2. *(A)* A close-up view of the gastroesophageal (GE) junction. *(B)* The lower esophageal sphincter (LES) is open. This position allows food and liquids to pass from the esophagus into the stomach but also allows stomach acid and other secretions to reflux up into the esophagus. *(C)* The LES is closed, preventing gastric secretions from refluxing up into the esophagus.

discussed later, we believe that pepsin may also play a role in both the development and the complications of GERD.

The Gastroesophageal Junction

The esophagus joins the stomach at an area called the *gastroesophageal junction,* or *GE junction* for short (see Figure 2.2). This area is important for several reasons. The first is the circular band of smooth muscle located at this junction. This ring of tissue, called the *lower esophageal sphincter* (LES), is about one and a half inches long and plays a pivotal role in preventing GERD (when it is functioning properly) and causing GERD (when it is not). A *sphincter* is any such muscular ring by which an opening of the body is normally kept closed. (Another ring of muscle is located at the top of the esophagus. This *upper esophageal sphincter* helps prevent acid from washing all the way up the esophagus into the mouth.)

In its normal position, the lower esophageal sphincter is contracted, or closed, to prevent food, liquid, and acid from regurgitating upward from the stomach into the esophagus. This prevents direct communication between the esophagus and stomach. Clearly, however, the sphincter must open to allow food or liquid to pass out of the esophagus into the stomach. Once the food or liquid has gone into the stomach, the LES normally tightens up again. Nevertheless, everyone's LES will from time to time relax enough to allow a small amount of acid to reflux, or splash back up, into the esophagus. This is called *physiologic reflux,* and most people never develop symptoms from it. Studies have shown that most people spend about 4 percent of their day (or about one hour each day) in physiologic reflux.

In some people, however, the LES is weak and does not contract properly, and in other people the LES contracts normally but relaxes too frequently. If the LES relaxes for too long, if it relaxes too frequently, or if it fails to close at all, then acid reflux is bound to occur, and GERD symptoms will almost certainly be produced.

The symptoms of GERD occur when the lining of the esophagus is irritated by acid (and possibly other chemicals). The esophagus has several defense mechanisms to protect it from irritation. First, acid that refluxes into the esophagus from the stomach is normally swept back into the stomach by the muscular contractions of the esophagus. Second, saliva helps to neutralize this acid. Finally, mucus also helps protect the esophagus from irritation. However, sometimes the amount of acid that refluxes is too great for the defense mechanisms of the esophagus, or the reflux happens so frequently that the esophagus cannot recover quickly enough. These episodes of acid coming into contact with the esophageal mucosa (the lining of the esophagus) can cause pain, the symptoms we diagnose as heartburn or GERD. Most of these episodes of esophageal contact with the acid last only seconds, but some episodes may last a few minutes (although the *symptoms* of the reflux may last much longer than the actual reflux).

In some people the symptoms of GERD persist well after the acid is no longer actually in contact with the esophagus, as they did for Joe after his celebratory dinner (see Chapter 1). Some people do not have *any* symptoms of GERD, however, although there may be hours each day when acid is in contact with the lining of their esophagus. This is one of the many reasons why GERD can be so difficult to diagnose. Prolonged contact of the esophagus with stomach acid can lead to permanent damage to the esophagus and complications that become apparent only later (see Chapter 8 for more information on complications).

The GE junction is also important because it is the junction between two critically different cell types that line the esophagus and the stomach. The innermost layer of the esophagus is covered with a cell type called *squamous epithelium;* these flat cells group together to form *squamous mucosa,* a lining that protects the more sensitive inner layers of the esophagus from stomach acid. The stomach is lined with a different type of cell, called *columnar epithelium;* these taller cells join together to form *columnar mucosa.* These two types of mucosa—squamous mucosa and columnar mucosa—meet at the GE junction and can easily be identified during endoscopy. Squamous and columnar mucosa differ greatly in their abilities to resist the harmful effects of stomach acid. The lining of the esophagus can be sensitive to even brief attacks by gastric acid, while the mucosa of the stomach is routinely bathed in acid and is rarely damaged by it (see plate 1, facing page 130).

Finally, the area of the GE junction is vulnerable in people who have had GERD for years, because a condition called *Barrett's esophagus* may develop here (see Chapter 8 for more details).

Fact or Fiction?

Now that we've described the physiology of GERD, we'd like to take a brief detour to put to rest three misconceptions about heartburn, or GERD. The first is that people with GERD have heartburn because they produce more stomach acid than people who do not suffer from GERD. This just isn't so, as several good studies have shown. People with GERD *do not* make more acid than people without GERD, and this is equally true whether the stomach is empty or full.

The real problem is not the amount of acid in the stomach per se, but the amount of acid that washes back up into the esophagus repeatedly, or acid that remains in the esophagus for too long. When we say that irritation occurs when the amount of acid that refluxes is too great for the defense mechanisms of the esophagus, we don't mean that an excess of stomach acid is *produced;* we mean that an excess of stomach acid is regurgitated into the esophagus.

Why does this misconception persist? One reason is that people know that many of the medications used to treat acid reflux act by reducing or eliminating stomach acid. But this does not mean that people with GERD produce more acid, it just means that suppressing acid production helps treat GERD symptoms. Although reducing stomach acid does not address the underlying reflux problem, episodes of gastric acid reflux are less damaging if the liquid refluxed into the esophagus is less acidic. Effective medications to correct a weakened or ineffective lower esophageal sphincter—one of the *real* main causes of GERD—are not yet available.

The second misconception about GERD is that acid is the only chemical that causes GERD. For many years physicians believed that only acid could cause GERD. However, there is now some information from laboratory and clinical studies to support the notion that other chemicals or agents, including bile and pepsin, may also play a role.

Bile is a liquid produced by the liver and stored in the gallbladder

Foods and Medications That Relax the Lower Esophageal Sphincter

Foods

Alcohol

Caffeine (coffee, cola, tea)

Chocolate

Licorice

Nicotine (cigarettes)

Peppermint

Spearmint

High-fat foods (cream, oils)

Medications

Anticholinergics

Barbiturates (for example, phenobarbital, secobarbital)

Calcium-channel blockers (diltiazem, nifedipine, verapamil)

Diazepam (brand name Valium)

Progesterone (for example, Prempro)

Prostaglandins

Sedatives (benzodiazepines)

Sumitriptan (migraine medicine, such as Imitrex)

Theophylline

until needed. Its function is to help digest fats by emulsifying them (breaking them into smaller fragments called *globules*). Bile from the liver can also mix with chemicals and secretions produced by the pancreas. These pancreatic juices contain digestive enzymes and an alkaline fluid containing bicarbonate. Bicarbonate helps to buffer or neutralize the acidic stomach juices.

While bile and pancreatic juices normally stay in the gallbladder and intestines, sometimes they mix together and reflux back into the stomach and from there into the esophagus, just like acid does. Some researchers and physicians believe that bile can be just as injurious to the esophagus as acid.

Pepsin is the active form of the precursor enzyme pepsinogen, which, as noted above, is secreted by cells lining the stomach and helps to digest protein. If pepsin refluxes into the esophagus, it can start to "digest" the proteins in the lining of the esophagus, particularly if that lining has already been damaged by acid reflux. So this, too, may play a role in injuring the esophagus.

A final misconception many people hold is that eating spicy foods or citrus or tomato products will cause heartburn. This is usually not the case, however. Contrary to popular opinion, spicy, citrus-based, and tomato-based foods do not directly cause heartburn, but they *can* irritate an esophagus that is already inflamed, and many people with GERD feel better if they avoid these foods.

On the other hand, research has clearly shown that specific foods, medications, and activities cause the LES to relax, and this, as explained above, can increase the chances that a person will develop heartburn. Many people have found that by simply eliminating some foods and activities, they can avoid heartburn altogether. Others have found that their GERD symptoms greatly improve if they avoid these food and activities.

If you are bothered by GERD symptoms, as a general rule you may want to avoid large meals and fatty or greasy foods, as well as the specific categories of foods and medications that relax the LES (see box, page 19). Chapter 5 provides more detail about how to make dietary changes and other lifestyle changes to prevent GERD.

Hiatal Hernia and GERD

Recall the following two anatomical details from earlier in this chapter: first, that the stomach normally lies beneath the diaphragm, and, second, that the esophagus passes from the chest cavity into the abdominal cavity through an opening in the diaphragm called the *esophageal hiatus*. If this opening in the diaphragm becomes wider than normal, then part of the stomach may slide up into the chest cavity from its normal position in the abdominal cavity. We call this condition a *hernia*. (A hernia is any swelling formed when part of an organ is displaced and protrudes through an opening in the wall of the body cavity normally containing the organ. Hernias can occur in many parts of the body, not just at the esophageal hiatus. A hernia around the belly button is called an *umbilical hernia,* and one in the groin may be either an *inguinal hernia* or a *femoral hernia.*)

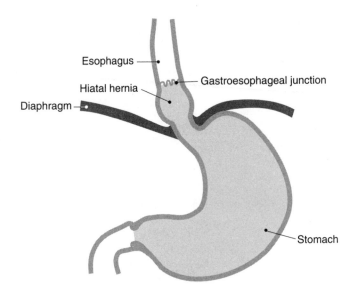

Figure 2.3. A hiatal hernia. Part of the stomach (usually the upper part, the *fundus*) has migrated from the abdominal cavity up into the chest cavity. Note how the GE junction has been displaced upward because of this.

There are two general types of stomach hernia. The most common is a *hiatal hernia*. A hiatal hernia occurs when a part of the stomach (usually the upper part) moves up through the esophageal hiatus and thus moves from the abdominal cavity into the thoracic cavity (see Figure 2.3). In a person with a hiatal hernia, the gastroesophageal junction is located above the level of the diaphragm rather than below, where it belongs. This change in position of the stomach can easily be seen endoscopically (through a fiberoptic tube), because the columnar mucosa of the stomach is higher than it should be. (Recall that the squamous mucosa of the esophagus and the columnar mucosa of the stomach meet at the GE junction.) Hiatal hernias can be locked into a set position, in which case they don't move. More commonly, however, the hernia can move, in which case it is said to be a *sliding hernia*—that is, the upper part of the stomach may freely slide from its normal position in the abdomen into the chest and back again.

The second type of stomach hernia is a *paraesophageal hernia*. In this type of hernia, the upper part of the stomach moves from the abdomi-

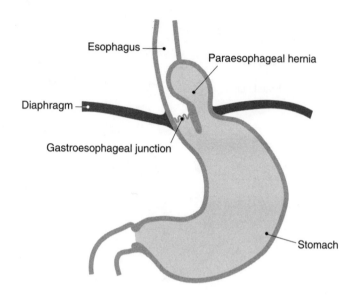

Figure 2.4. A paraesophageal hernia. Part of the stomach has moved from the abdominal cavity up into the thoracic cavity. In contrast to what happens with a hiatal hernia, the GE junction here has not changed position and remains at the level of the diaphragm.

nal cavity into the thoracic cavity. Most commonly, the hernia occurs anterior to (in front of) the esophagus. In this case, the gastroesophageal junction retains its normal location at the esophageal hiatus of the diaphragm (see Figure 2.4), because what moves up into the thoracic cavity is part of the stomach that does not include the GE junction. Paraesophageal hernias, which are much less common than hiatal hernias, usually cause pain, difficulty swallowing, or (less often) a choking sensation or a feeling of shortness of breath.

Some people are born with a hernia, and in this case the hernia, wherever it is located, is said to be *congenital* (existing from birth but not hereditary). Most hiatal hernias develop as people get older, however, and some researchers estimate that 40 to 50 percent of people over age 50 have one. Hernias in people over the age of 50 may occur because of the natural weakening of muscle tone with age. Repetitive lifting and straining, however, which puts stress on the muscle fibers around the esophageal hiatus, can also cause these muscle fibers to become looser and to widen and can contribute to the development of a hernia.

What about the symptoms of hiatal hernia? Many people believe that hiatal hernias cause pain, swallowing problems, belching, burping, or gassiness. In fact, most people who have a hiatal hernia have no symptoms and are never even aware that they have one. Because they do not notice anything amiss, they may never consult a physician and will never know they have a hiatal hernia unless they undergo testing for some reason, such as gastrointestinal symptoms. A person with gastrointestinal symptoms may see a physician for diagnosis and treatment of these symptoms, and if an x-ray study (i.e., barium swallow) or endoscopy is part of the diagnostic examination, the person may be diagnosed as having a hiatal hernia at the same time he or she is diagnosed with GERD or another ailment.

The two most accurate tests for diagnosing a hiatal hernia are an upper endoscopy (EGD) and an x-ray study such as a barium swallow or upper gastrointestinal series (upper GI series). (See Chapter 4 for a description of these tests.)

Although a hiatal hernia will not cause GERD, it can make GERD symptoms worse, especially if the hernia is large. Acid washing back up into the esophagus from the stomach may become trapped in the hernia sac for long periods, and this can cause persistent irritation. In addition, a hiatal hernia prevents the esophagus from contracting normally, a process that routinely occurs to empty the esophagus of saliva, mucus, and any acid that may have refluxed up from the stomach. As noted above, if the esophagus fails to contract normally, acid can remain in the esophagus for prolonged periods and produce irritation and inflammation. This condition is called *esophagitis*. This process may become a vicious circle, because once esophagitis develops, the lower esophageal sphincter does not contract as well, more acid refluxes, and the inflammation caused by chronic acid exposure gets worse.

Hiatal hernias that do not cause symptoms do not need to be repaired. But if someone is having surgery to treat GERD (for example, because his or her GERD cannot be treated adequately with medications), then if a hiatal hernia is present, it is usually repaired at the same time.

It is important to stress that paraesophageal hernias are different from hiatal hernias in this respect. Paraesophageal hernias usually *do* cause symptoms, and they are much more likely to lead to complications such as bleeding or even strangulation. Therefore, paraesophageal hernias should almost always be repaired surgically.

Finally, when a hernia is strangulated, the blood supply is cut off, and as a result the tissue may die. A *strangulated hernia,* wherever it occurs, must be surgically repaired, usually on an emergency basis. This is rare with hiatal hernias.

In the next part of the book we'll take a closer look at the symptoms of GERD and the steps taken in diagnosing the disorder, beginning, in Chapter 3, with common—and not so common—symptoms.

Part II

SYMPTOMS
& DIAGNOSIS

What Are the Symptoms of GERD?

Remember Joe? In Chapter 1 we said that Joe's symptoms, and how they progressed and responded to treatment, were typical of GERD. In this chapter we'll take a much closer look at these symptoms, beginning with the most common and moving on to the less typical and even the rare ways in which GERD can "declare itself." This information may help you understand any symptoms you may be experiencing, and it will help you understand GERD better.

Before we get into specifics about symptoms, however, three important points need to be made. First, absence of symptoms is not a guarantee of absence of GERD. In Chapter 2 we noted that many people do not have *any* symptoms of heartburn, even though acid is in contact with their esophagus for hours each day. While we don't know how many people have *asymptomatic GERD* (GERD that is present without any symptoms), some experts estimate that up to one-third of people who later develop problems from acid reflux never have any symptoms from it. Thus, it is not uncommon to have a patient tell his or her doctor about swallowing difficulties and then find out that the difficulties are due to chronic esophagitis that has caused a stricture (narrowing) at the lower end of the esophagus. Yet the patient was never bothered by symptoms like heartburn. We know that GERD-related strictures (called *peptic strictures,* because they are caused by stomach acid) do not develop quickly. If someone develops a peptic stricture in the absence of symptoms, then stomach acid must have been quietly refluxing into the esophagus for quite some time, probably years.

Still more common is this scenario: a patient is evaluated by a gastroenterologist for non-GERD symptoms, such as abdominal pain or blood loss, and the physician finds evidence of esophagitis during the endoscopy, even though the person has never had any symptoms of heartburn or regurgitation. Doctors do not normally perform an upper endoscopy or a 24-hour pH test (another test for GERD, described in Chapter 4) on people who do not have symptoms of GERD, and so it is difficult to say whether or not any one particular person is likely to have GERD in the absence of symptoms. What is clear is that some people have GERD without any symptoms, and these individuals are nonetheless at risk of developing some of the complications of GERD described in Chapter 8.

Does this mean that everyone should be evaluated by endoscopy for evidence of GERD? No. Even aside from the logistical and cost considerations of scheduling millions of endoscopies, GERD is by and large a benign disease. In addition, looking for GERD in people who have no symptoms would cause more problems than would result if we evaluated or tested only those people who *do* have symptoms. (One reason we can't simply test everyone for GERD is that a small number of people would suffer a complication from the upper endoscopy or 24-hour pH testing needed to diagnose GERD, and these real risks would outweigh the potential benefits of looking for GERD in everyone.)

The second important general point about GERD symptoms is that symptom severity is not a good predictor of the severity of GERD or the likelihood of a person developing complications like esophagitis or strictures. A patient who has few or no symptoms of GERD may develop complications, while a patient with ongoing discomfort from symptoms of GERD may have little or no physical damage or complications. This is very frustrating for physicians and patients alike. Even so, people who have acid reflux but don't have symptoms are generally less likely to have active, destructive disease than people who have symptomatic acid reflux. Still, we need to keep in mind that some people with no symptoms or mild symptoms do nevertheless have significant disease. Two examples will illustrate.

First, consider Joe. Initially, if you'll recall, his heartburn symptoms responded well to antacids and H_2-blockers. Yet these treatments did not halt the persistent damage being done to his esophagus by stomach acid. We learned this when Joe underwent endoscopy as his symptoms got worse and he was found to have ongoing esophagitis. In Joe's case, the treatments *appeared* to be working well because the symptoms disappeared, but the *actual reflux of acid into the esophagus*—the hallmark of GERD—continued to occur and caused the esophagitis to get worse.

A second example is almost any older person with GERD. Both older men and older women complain less about heartburn than younger people do. One might assume from this that older people are less likely to have GERD, and that they perhaps have milder disease when they do have GERD. The opposite is true, however. Older people (in this context, usually defined as those over age 60) are *more* likely to have GERD and tend to have *greater* acid reflux and *more* injury to their esophagus than younger people with GERD.

Why, then, do older people report less severe symptoms? The answer may lie in a difference in pain perception between older and younger individuals. Studies have shown that when a small balloon is gradually filled with air in the esophagus of volunteers, younger people without GERD find the procedure uncomfortable or painful sooner than older people without GERD. That is, the younger people feel discomfort when the balloon is smaller, but many older people don't have a sense of discomfort until the balloon is larger. In another study, when dilute acid was dripped into the esophagus of volunteers who were known to have GERD, on average it took longer for older people to perceive that they were experiencing heartburn, and they perceived their symptoms as less severe than did the younger people with GERD. What this means is that older individuals form a group who may have more severe disease than their symptoms suggest, and they should be evaluated and treated more aggressively. The potential severity of their disease should not be underestimated.

The third point to make at the beginning of this chapter on symptoms is that there is a fair amount of overlap between what we call *symptoms* and what we call *complications*. An increase in the wheezing of asthma may be a *symptom* of underlying gastroesophageal reflux disease, for example. But when the wheezing is so bad that the person can't run, or lands in the emergency room once a month, then we may consider the worsening of asthma to be a *complication* of GERD. Complications in the esophagus such as esophagitis and Barrett's esophagus are covered in Chapter 8 of this book. In this chapter we look at symptoms, including those that develop in areas other than the esophagus. The reader should be aware, however, that persistent or severe symptoms may also be considered complications of acid reflux disease.

Common Symptoms of GERD

As noted in Chapter 1, the most common symptoms of GERD are heartburn and regurgitation. *Heartburn* (also called *pyrosis*) is experienced by most people at some time or another. It requires evaluation by a specialist only when it is experienced repeatedly, when it persists despite over-the-counter remedies, or when it is accompanied by more alarming symptoms such as weight loss, difficulty swallowing, or bleeding. If you've never experienced heartburn, it may be difficult to imagine what it feels like—and if you have, you're painfully familiar with this unpleasant sensation. Most people describe it as a burning, dull ache, pain, or discomfort behind the sternum (breastbone), often seeming to extend up in the chest, occasionally as far up as the throat. The discomfort of heartburn can be so intense that it feels like a heart attack, or so mild that it's barely noticeable.

Heartburn tends to (but does not necessarily) occur after a meal, and especially after a large meal eaten at night or a meal that includes fatty foods, alcohol, caffeine, chocolate, or peppermint. What else can cause GERD symptoms? Any of the following, alone or in combination:

* vigorous exercise
* tight clothing

* lying down after eating any kind of food
* smoking
* bending over
* coughing
* being overweight or obese

By the way, having a big belly for any reason can cause heartburn symptoms. Besides obesity, the most common causes of an abnormally large belly are pregnancy or abnormal fluid in the abdominal cavity. (Abnormal fluid in the abdominal cavity, a condition called *ascites*, is usually related to excessive alcohol consumption over many years, but it can also be caused by cancer or hepatitis.)

Many of the items on this list lead to stomach acid refluxing into the esophagus either because they affect the stomach or because they affect the lower esophageal sphincter. Obesity, tight clothing, bending over, and coughing tend to increase pressure in the abdomen so that stomach contents are forced upward. Fatty foods, chocolate, and smoking, on the other hand, cause heartburn by reducing the pressure in the LES, thereby reducing its effectiveness as a mechanical barrier to the upward movement of stomach acid. Additionally, there are medications, such as some asthma medicines, that have the side effect of reducing LES pressure.

Another common symptom of GERD is acid *regurgitation,* which is the sensation that occurs when acid travels all the way up from the stomach, past both the lower and upper esophageal sphincters, into the mouth. Many people have experienced the sour taste in the mouth caused by regurgitation. In an effort to clear the acid that is refluxing, many people swallow repeatedly; but this results in air being swallowed along with saliva. This swallowing of air can produce gaseous distention of the stomach and the GERD symptom of *excessive belching.* Repeated belching brings up even more acid, in a vicious cycle of acid reflux, air swallowing, and belching.

When acid is refluxed into the esophagus, the salivary glands may produce large volumes of alkaline (bicarbonate-rich) foamy or frothy secretions in an attempt to neutralize the stomach acid. Because of the amount of saliva involved and the suddenness with which it appears in the mouth, this phenomenon, called *water brash,* can be startling. The saliva in water brash may taste slightly salty. A case example is useful in demonstrating this symptom.

Lorraine, a 76-year-old retiree, was referred to Dr. Evan Strayer for a second opinion regarding her "swallowing difficulties." She arrived at Dr. Strayer's office impeccably dressed and regally composed except for one small detail. In her left hand she carried a large red cup into which she would spit every five minutes or so. She said she had been carrying the cup for the past two years because her mouth continually filled up with fluid, and she could not swallow it fast enough to keep it from spilling out of her mouth. She was embarrassed by this, of course, but the cup was the only way she could go out in public without continually visiting a rest room to spit the fluid from her mouth.

Lorraine's family doctor was concerned that she might have a stricture of the esophagus, or even cancer of the esophagus, and he had ordered a barium swallow to look for a blockage or stricture. The test results were completely normal, but Lorraine's doctor still had concerns, and he asked Lorraine to see a specialist in swallowing disorders, a gastroenterologist. The gastroenterologist saw her and recommended that she have an upper endoscopy, which, again, was normal. Lorraine continued to have problems swallowing her saliva, however, and her doctors were stumped, so Dr. Strayer, a specialist in gastroesophageal disorders, was asked to see her.

Dr. Strayer began by asking Lorraine if she had ever had symptoms of heartburn. She emphatically said no—she could eat whatever she wanted and never had to take over-the-counter antacids. She denied suffering from regurgitation or heartburn. After taking Lorraine's life history and examining her, Dr. Strayer began to suspect that her symptom was water brash. Lorraine was skeptical, because she never had heartburn or an acid taste in her mouth. Dr. Strayer recommended that she try a two-week course of lansoprazole, a potent acid-suppressing medication of the proton-pump inhibitor type, to see if her symptoms improved. (This approach—treating a presumed illness to find out whether the treatment takes care of the symptoms—is called a *therapeutic trial.*) Lorraine did not want to take pills that she thought were not necessary, and she declined the suggested therapeutic trial of antacids. She did, however, agree to a 24-hour pH probe (see Chapter 4) to determine whether acid reflux was occurring and to measure the extent of acid reflux over a full day and night. Dr. Strayer asked

Lorraine to keep a record during the 24-hour period of when her mouth filled up with fluid, so that he could correlate these episodes with any acid reflux she might have.

Although not surprising to Dr. Strayer, the result of the 24-hour pH probe was surprising to Lorraine. During much of the day and night she had multiple and prolonged episodes of acid refluxing up into her esophagus. Many of these episodes correlated perfectly to her water brash—the times when her mouth filled up with frothy secretions. Dr. Strayer explained that this was not uncommon and that many people have significant acid reflux and do not feel it as heartburn. Now that there was objective data in hand, Lorraine agreed to a trial of lansoprazole for a month.

When Lorraine returned to see Dr. Strayer, she was as well groomed as ever, but this time she came without the red cup. Appearing greatly relieved, she told Dr. Strayer she had seen a remarkable improvement over the last two weeks, that she was now able to swallow all of her secretions easily. Dr. Strayer asked her to decrease the dose of her proton-pump inhibitor to once a day, and when he saw her three months later she again arrived without complaints—and without the cup.

While heartburn, regurgitation, and water brash are considered the classic symptoms of GERD, a less common but also typical symptom of GERD involves *swallowing difficulties*. Some people feel as if they are having trouble swallowing at all, and some people feel pain when they swallow. When people visit their doctors because they are having difficulty swallowing (called *dysphagia*), doctors often discover, in the course of doing tests to find out what's causing the difficulty, that the person has chronic esophagitis from GERD that has caused a stricture of the lower end of the esophagus. It is logical to think that if a person is having trouble swallowing, then the stricture would be located at the throat end of the esophagus, but in fact a stricture that high up in the esophagus is extremely uncommon. This is because acid would have to splash up very high to form a stricture at the level of the throat (remember that the esophagus is 10 inches long). Acid reflux usually occurs right at the junction of the esophagus and the stomach, so what actually happens is this: Because of how the nerves in the esophagus send messages, where you feel distress (in the throat) is often not where the stricture is located (although sometimes it is). The stricture located at the lower esophageal junction may cause a tightening in your throat and a feeling that food sticks, or catches. (Feeling or sensing pain in one area when the problem or abnormality causing the pain is located somewhere else is called *referred pain.*)

Difficulty swallowing, particularly in an older individual, is an alarming symptom that can indicate a serious underlying condition such as cancer of the esophagus. *Anyone who experiences difficult or painful swallowing should undergo evaluation* by a gastroenterologist. Such an evaluation would include an upper endoscopy or an upper GI series of x-rays.

Chest Pain

When people with GERD experience chest pain that is more severe than the typically mild or moderate degree of pain experienced as heartburn, the pain may be caused by a spasm (strong contraction) of the esophagus. This intense pain may make it more difficult to distinguish GERD pain from cardiac pain, but in truth it is often difficult for people to distinguish between the chest pain of heartburn, on the one hand, and chest pain from one of two conditions in the heart, on the other hand. The chest pain resulting from reduced blood flow to the heart, called *angina pectoris,* is one heart condition; the other is a *myocardial infarction,* more commonly known as a *heart attack,* which is caused by severely reduced or interrupted blood flow to a portion of the heart that results in death of a portion of the heart muscle. The pain of heartburn and the pain of heart attack are probably easily mistaken for each other because the heart and the esophagus share a common system of nerves. The heart and the esophagus are also neighbors in the chest. While people who have experienced both heart-related chest pain and heartburn can usually distinguish the source of the pain or discomfort, someone experiencing a single episode of one or the other may have difficulty telling them apart. And of course *anyone*— including anyone with GERD—can have a heart attack.

The bottom line is that it is crucially important not to disregard the signs of a heart attack by brushing them off as an attack of painful acid reflux. If the opposite occurs, and the pain of acid reflux is mistaken for a heart attack, probably the worst thing that will happen is an unnecessary ride in an ambulance or visit to the emergency room. To avoid mistakenly assuming that chest pain is GERD when it is something more serious, the rule of thumb is that *any chest pain that is not typical heartburn pain and familiar to the individual experiencing it should be assumed to be cardiac in origin until proven otherwise.*

What happens when someone is taken to the hospital complaining of chest pain? The hospital's priority is to properly evaluate the chest pain and determine what's causing it. This includes quickly ruling out the possibility that the pain is cardiac in origin. Tests to determine injury to the heart include electrocardiograms (EKGs), blood tests for the enzymes that are secreted in response to damage to the heart muscle, and exercise stress-testing with or without nuclear medicine studies (for example, a stress thallium test). *Esophageal motility testing* is occasionally performed to evaluate chest pain. For this test, a thin, flexible tube for measuring pressures in the esophagus is inserted through the nose, down the esophagus, and into the stomach. Esophageal motility testing may reveal that the source of the chest pain is related to an *esophageal motility disorder.* (This test would be performed not in the emergency room but at a later date, once it was clear that the pain was not due to a heart problem.)

Esophageal motility disorders are conditions that impair the normal movement of ingested liquids and solids down the esophagus into the stomach. Many of these conditions can cause chest pain, but the chest pain is *noncardiac* in origin (rather than being related to the heart, the pain is due to something else). The three esophageal motility disorders causing chest pain that are most commonly identified through testing are:

* the so-called *nutcracker esophagus,* in which the inside of the esophagus contracts at very high pressures;
* *diffuse esophageal spasm,* a condition of periodic clamping down of the esophagus, in many cases brought about by swallowing; and

* *nonspecific esophageal motility disorder,* a term for poorly understood abnormalities in esophageal pressures or abnormalities in the propagation of waves of pressure moving down the esophagus that do not fall into a well-defined constellation of findings.

These conditions are usually unrelated to GERD and are treated differently from GERD. Different medications are used, for example, including nitrates to reduce esophageal pressures.

To summarize: while is usually possible to distinguish cardiac pain from GERD-related chest pain, it is best to seek medical help immediately if (1) you have any doubts or (2) even if you are convinced that the pain is heartburn, the pain does not respond to treatment that has helped in the past.

Lung Symptoms

Many people are surprised to learn that GERD can affect or injure other parts of the body besides the esophagus, but it can. The lungs, for example, are commonly affected by acid reflux. Acid can enter the lungs by first refluxing into the pharynx and from there traveling to the lungs. Stomach acid can alter lung function, and acid reflux is responsible for several different problems in the lungs. One of the most common is asthma. Other common problems include chronic cough, chronic bronchitis, aspiration pneumonia, interstitial pulmonary fibrosis, and possibly a sleep disturbance called sleep apnea. Aspiration of acid and other gastric contents into the lung can produce fever, cough, shortness of breath, an elevated white count, and chest x-ray findings similar to what you would see with bacterial pneumonia, but in *aspiration pneumonia* the culprits are not bacteria. *Pulmonary fibrosis* is a condition that develops in response to chronic injury and inflammation in the lung. Fibrosis prevents the lungs from expanding fully, and this causes people to become short of breath. *Sleep apnea* is a condition in which the person has brief spells of not breathing during sleep. It is characterized by snoring, disordered sleep, and extreme sleepiness during the day.

Asthma

Asthma is a disorder of the lungs in which the airways are overly reactive to various stimuli. When the airways are hyperreactive, they may constrict (a condition called *bronchoconstriction*) and become quite narrowed, which can make breathing difficult. In addition, during an asthma attack, the *bronchioles,* or small breathing tubes, become swollen and inflamed. This leads to further narrowing of the airways, which can make breathing difficult, even when the person is resting.

Acid in the esophagus can produce asthma or make it worse in one of two ways. Either one or both of these mechanisms may play a role in the development or perpetuation of an asthma attack. In the first, the *reflux mechanism,* the person inhales, or *aspirates,* tiny quantities of acid from the esophagus into the lungs via the windpipe; this inhalation of microscopic particles is called *microaspiration* (see Figure 3.1 *[A]*). Stomach acid is at least as irritating to the lungs and passageways leading to the lungs as it is to the lining of the esophagus, and the body's response to this irritation is a swelling *(edema)* and reflex narrowing or spasm of the passageways into the lungs *(bronchospasm).*

This swelling and narrowing causes wheezing, particularly at night, after lying down. When a person is lying down it is easier for stomach acid to find its way into the lungs, because the acid does not have to fight gravity to make its way to the back of the throat. Wheezing is sometimes hardly noticeable, but sometimes it is severe enough to be life-threatening. In wheezing, the breathing sounds are louder than usual, and they often have a musical quality that can be heard by other people. The stethoscopes used by physicians help them hear the breathing sounds through the person's back. Wheezing is the primary symptom of asthma.

The second way in which acid in the esophagus can produce asthma is via what is called the *reflex mechanism.* Here, gastric acid acts as an irritant to the nerves that supply the esophagus. These nerves (primarily branches of the vagus nerve) also send signals to the lungs, and when they are irritated, they tell the breathing passages in the lung to

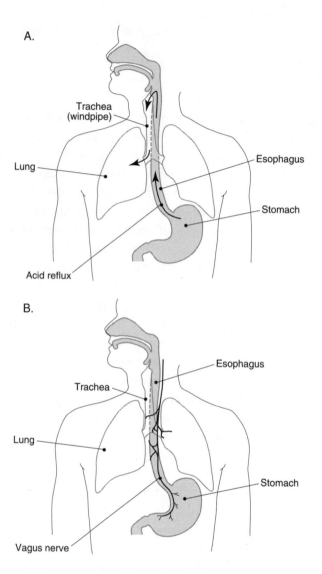

Figure 3.1. *(A)* Acid can reflux from the stomach directly up the esophagus into the trachea (windpipe) and then travel from the trachea into the lung. This reflux may produce irritation and inflammation, leading to chronic cough, asthma, and laryngitis. *(B)* Acid that refluxes into the lower end of the esophagus stimulates chemical receptors located in the mucosa. When these receptors are stimulated, messages are transmitted through the vagus nerve, and then the person may have a cough, begin wheezing, or have a constant need to clear the throat.

contract (see Figure 3.1 *[B]*). In this case, GERD can lead to wheezing even if stomach acid does not reflux all the way into the lungs, because the esophagus and the lung passageways share a common origin during fetal development in the womb, so that when the nerves of the esophagus are irritated by acid, there is a reflex irritation of the lung passageways, resulting in spasm and wheezing.

The connection between GERD and asthma was not apparent to doctors and researchers at first, partly because both of these diseases are very common. It is estimated that more than 20 million Americans have asthma and, as we have noted, that as many as 60 million Americans have GERD. So when a person has both GERD and asthma, it is logical to conclude that this is coincidental. Eventually, however, several good medical studies demonstrated that when a patient has both conditions at the same time, it is usually more than just a coincidence. These studies have shown that a large proportion of patients with asthma suffer from persistent GERD symptoms (43 to 82 percent, depending on the study). While it seems that this bronchospasm occurs in all people to some extent when acid refluxes into the esophagus, it is more pronounced, and does not clear as quickly, in people with asthma. Therefore, when a person is having a medical evaluation for wheezing, GERD should be suspected as a cause of the wheezing, particularly in individuals who began wheezing for the first time as adults (because asthma more typically begins in childhood) and in individuals whose wheezing is not brought on or made worse by physical exertion or exposure to allergens (dust, mold, etc.).

Medical studies have also revealed that treating heartburn aggressively with medications can have many benefits in people with asthma. These benefits may include a reduction in the need for steroids (usually prednisone), a decrease in the number of medications or in the dose of medications needed to control asthma, an increase in the ability to exercise, and an overall improvement in breathing.

People who have both asthma and classic symptoms of GERD do not require any special tests and can be treated with H_2-blockers (cimetidine, famotidine, nizatidine, or ranitidine) or proton-pump inhibitors (omeprazole, lansoprazole, rabeprazole, esomeprazole, pantoprazole). There is no indication that one type of drug is clearly better than another at the beginning. The choice of medication for *any* patient should be based on several considerations, including eliminating symptoms, healing esophagitis (if present), maintaining the esophagus in a healed state (once healed), and preventing complications.

One important point brought out by studies in patients with asthma and GERD is that the beneficial effects of the GERD medicines are not always immediately apparent. For some patients, an improvement in asthma symptoms may not be noticed for three months or more, and seeing improvement often means taking fairly high doses of medication. In our practice, if we are concerned that a patient's asthma is the result of chronic acid reflux, we usually treat that patient aggressively for at least three months with a twice-a-day proton-pump inhibitor. (See Chapters 6 and 7 for a complete discussion of GERD medications.)

Finally, some patients with severe asthma and severe GERD may find that medications such as proton-pump inhibitors help but do not completely eliminate symptoms of heartburn, and that their asthma does not improve as much as they and their doctor had hoped. This is a reminder that asthma is often the result of multiple factors. Unless these other factors are also treated, treating only the GERD will most likely not entirely clear up the problem. People with asthma who do not get complete relief of symptoms when they take medications for acid reflux find that they must take the medications continuously in order to keep their asthma symptoms at bay. Patients in both of these categories—insufficient asthma relief or chronic use of GERD medications—may be candidates for surgery to alleviate their heartburn symptoms. This will make it easier for such patients to address some of the other factors causing their asthma, in the first case, and to discontinue GERD medications, in the second.

Heartburn can make asthma worse. But can asthma make heartburn worse? Yes, although this effect is much less common than the opposite one. As noted above, one way asthma can affect GERD is through the medications, called *bronchodilators*, that are used to treat asthma; these medications also reduce pressure in the lower esophageal sphincter and therefore increase the chance that acid will reflux up into the esophagus and cause problems. Another drug, theophylline, can also reduce LES pressure and increase the likelihood of reflux. Also, in some people with severe asthma, the anatomy of the lungs and that of the diaphragm undergo changes due to a process called *air trapping*. These changes may also change the anatomy of the gastroesophageal junction in a way that increases the chance of acid reflux.

Cough

A chronic cough that doesn't improve with antibiotics can also be a sign of GERD.

Jessamyn is 64 years old and considers herself to be in good health, other than having mild arthritis of the knees and being slightly overweight. But then she developed a cough. It occurred mostly at night and occasionally kept her awake for several hours. She did not bring up any phlegm or sputum, and she did not have any fevers, chills, or sweats at night. At first she thought the cough might be due to her cigarettes: she smoked three or four a day, usually at midday and while playing cards at night. She gave up even these few cigarettes, but her cough did not improve. For the next two months she tried different cough syrups, lozenges, and antihistamines, also without success.

Jessamyn finally went to see her doctor, who examined her nose, ears, mouth, neck, heart, lungs, and abdomen and found them to be normal. The doctor asked her if she ever had heartburn, and Jessamyn was pleased to say no. The doctor told her she probably had a virus or some irritation from her cigarettes, but just to be on the safe side she ordered a blood count and a chest x-ray. Both of these were normal. The cough persisted, although Jessamyn did not have any other symptoms. Her doctor tried her on prescription-strength antihistamines, nasal steroids, and even several different types of inhaled medications (puffers), thinking that Jessamyn's symptoms might be due to asthma. None of the medications worked.

Eight months after the cough started, Jessamyn's primary care doctor sent her to an ear, nose, and throat (ENT) doctor, who reported that the nose and ears looked perfectly normal but wondered whether there was some inflammation around the vocal cords—although Jessamyn had told her that she hadn't noticed a change in her voice. X-rays of the sinuses were taken and appeared normal. The ENT doctor suggested various types of medications to treat postnasal drip, and Jessamyn tried them for the next eight weeks—frustratingly, without relief.

When the ENT doctor recommended that Jessamyn see Dr. Amy Snead, a specialist in diagnosing and treating GERD, Jessamyn had had a persistent cough for more than 10 months. She told Dr. Snead that she could eat "anything" and never get heartburn. She did occasionally eat large meals at night, or have evening snacks, but this didn't bother her. She drank decaffeinated coffee at night, but she did not drink any alcohol, and she tried to avoid chocolate because of her weight. She never used any type of over-the-counter antacid. Dr. Snead told Jessamyn that she thought her chronic cough might be due to GERD, and she suggested a trial of a medicine to suppress gastric acid. Jessamyn was hesitant, because she "never" had heartburn and because she had already tried so many different medications without relief. She agreed to a month-long trial of omeprazole twice a day, however, and when she returned to see Dr. Snead a month later, she said that after about two weeks on the omeprazole her cough had improved greatly, and that in the last five days she had been "cough-free" for the first time in 10 months. Her only question was whether she could get a refill on her prescription.

It took a long time for the source of Jessamyn's cough to be diagnosed and treated, but this is not unusual, because evaluating a persistent cough can be very difficult. A cough that persists for more than three weeks is defined as *chronic* and is very different from an *acute* cough, which lasts only a few days or a week.

Cigarette smoking, postnasal drip, respiratory tract infections, and some medications are all common causes of chronic cough. Another cause of chronic cough is asthma, which, as we have seen, is sometimes made worse by GERD. A very common cause of chronic cough, however, is GERD itself, accounting in one study for 21 percent of cases of chronic cough. People with chronic cough due to GERD may cough only at night—but then, so may people with chronic cough due to postnasal drip.

People with a chronic cough and no history of heartburn, like Jessamyn, are difficult to diagnose. Remember that up to one-third of patients with GERD don't have heartburn; their only symptom of GERD may be a cough. A 24-hour pH probe is the best test to use to look for pulmonary symptoms (cough, wheezing, asthma flare) caused by acid reflux, although an upper endoscopy may also be helpful (see Chapter 4). The pH probe can measure the number of times, and the amount of time, that acid refluxes into the esophagus. In addition, this test can compare periods of acid reflux with episodes of coughing, to determine whether there is a connection between the two events.

To diagnose the underlying cause of a chronic cough, a physician may do any of the specific tests for asthma or GERD, or the physician may simply try treatment for the suspected cause of the chronic cough. For example, if antihistamines are used, chronic cough related to postnasal drip usually improves, while chronic cough related to asthma or GERD does not. A 12-week trial of a powerful antacid medication, usually one of the proton-pump inhibitors (omeprazole, lansoprazole, rabeprazole, esomeprazole, or pantoprazole, described in Chapter 7), will improve about half the cases of chronic cough in people who also have GERD.

Why not 100 percent improvement, if the chronic cough is caused by GERD? There are several possible explanations, more than one of which is likely to be playing a role. First, not all GERD responds to standard doses of a proton-pump inhibitor. Some people who do not respond to proton-pump inhibitor treatment fall into this category, and taking a higher dose of the proton-pump inhibitor will control the GERD-related cough for some of them. Second, there may be more than one cause of the chronic cough, and a proton-pump inhibitor might not cover the entire picture. Third, *not all associations are causation.* This is a common problem in medicine. A person can have both GERD and chronic cough and the cough will not respond even to effective treatment and control of the acid reflux. This may be because the cough is habitual—that is, the patient now coughs out of habit rather than because of any mechanical irritation of the pharynx. So, again, when GERD is properly treated, more than half, but not all, of the people with chronic cough due to GERD will stop coughing.

Many patients with chronic cough caused by GERD get complete relief of their cough by taking an H_2-blocker each night before going to bed. Others may need to take higher doses of H_2-blockers, proton-pump inhibitors, or even a combination of a proton-pump inhibitor during the day and ranitidine at night to eliminate their cough.

GERD Symptoms in the Head and Neck

Laryngitis that doesn't go away or ongoing hoarseness can be signs of persistent GERD. Some studies have shown that as many as 25 percent of people with GERD have only head and neck symptoms rather than any of the classic heartburn symptoms. The head and neck symptoms of GERD include:

* hoarseness
* persistent sore throat
* chronic throat clearing
* the sensation of a lump in the throat
* postnasal drip
* laryngitis
* vocal cord polyps
* a change in voice
* dental erosions
* severe bad breath
* chronic ear pain

These symptoms respond very well to treatment of GERD. In fact, they respond so well that if a patient is treated for GERD and these symptoms go away, then it is seldom necessary to search for other causes of the head and neck symptoms. Seeing an improvement is good evidence that GERD was, indeed, responsible for the symptoms.

How does GERD lead to this variety of seemingly unrelated head and neck symptoms? Studies indicate that direct acid damage is the most likely cause of these symptoms. The pharynx (the back of the throat) is directly connected to the esophagus, while the larynx (the voice box) contains the opening to the windpipe and the lungs, and also contains the vocal cords, which are responsible for producing speech. The esophagus, pharynx, and larynx are all close together, which is why it is so easy to inhale a bit of food or liquid when you actually mean to swallow it. It is also why symptoms of GERD can show up in the larynx and the pharynx. For example, acid reflux into the back of the throat can damage the larynx. Most of the damage seems to occur when the person has intermittent reflux while lying down at night.

Hoarseness is perhaps the best-studied head and neck symptom that may be related to GERD, yet treating the GERD does not always eliminate the hoarseness. Studies show that almost four out of five people with chronic hoarseness and other symptoms suggestive of GERD have abnormal 24-hour pH studies. However, about half of people who have chronic hoarseness with *or* without other symptoms suggestive of GERD also have abnormal 24-hour pH studies. Again, the most reasonable and helpful approach is usually a therapeutic trial with a proton-pump inhibitor to see whether the hoarseness improves.

When someone has chronic hoarseness, an ear, nose, and throat specialist may perform a test called *indirect laryngoscopy* to look at the throat and vocal cords for signs of acid damage or other conditions. Acid damage may also lead to chronic laryngitis and a persistent sore throat, as well. If a person has any of these symptoms and they are not controlled by treatment for GERD, the ENT specialist may detect redness of the vocal cords or the areas near them, or benign growths on the vocal cords such as polyps. Such findings, while abnormal, are seen not only when acid irritates this region but also when a person is a chronic smoker, abuses alcohol, abuses his or her voice (as some singers do), or has asthma or allergies. Again, a therapeutic trial may be necessary to get a better sense of what is likely causing the symptom or abnormal findings on indirect laryngoscopy.

Overall, to discover that chronic lung or head and neck symptoms are caused by GERD rather than by the more typical causes of these symptoms, a "high index of suspicion" is needed. That is, the doctor must *think* of GERD in order to *detect* it. This can be difficult when there are no obvious clues such as typical heartburn symptoms. Yet it is

something that physicians who treat GERD learn to think about, because GERD does, indeed, make itself known in a variety of ways—but
a known variety of ways.

Once GERD is suspected, a combination of therapeutic trials and
tests can confirm (or refute) the diagnosis of GERD, whether the
person has typical or unusual symptoms. In the next chapter we describe these therapeutic trials and tests in more detail.

Chapter 4

Diagnosing GERD

Some medical conditions or diseases are easy to identify. A doctor can diagnose high cholesterol, for example, through a simple blood test. And he or she can easily diagnose some types of rashes or fungal infections of the skin simply by looking at them and then confirming the diagnosis by examining scrapings of the skin under a microscope. Many infections of the urinary tract, too, can be diagnosed simply by listening to the patient describe symptoms and following up with a urinalysis and urine culture.

Gastroesophageal reflux disease, however, can be very difficult to diagnose. Here's why: although the basic *process* of GERD is essentially the same in every person who suffers from this condition (stomach acid refluxing into the esophagus), different people *experience* this process in different ways, ranging from mild heartburn to a variety of more distressing symptoms to no symptoms at all. The variety of symptoms, and the different ways people experience them, in part explains why it is sometimes difficult to diagnose GERD.

Many people with acid reflux disease have what are considered characteristic or classic symptoms: *Heartburn*—a burning sensation beneath the breastbone that may radiate up into the throat or mouth. *Regurgitation*—the unexpected movement of small amounts of fluid or food from the stomach back into the esophagus and mouth. *Water brash*—the sudden filling up of the mouth with frothy or foamy liquid. This last condition is due to the sudden and rapid release of saliva into the mouth in response to acid reflux. The saliva is produced in an attempt to neutralize the acid and thus protect the esophagus.

When these classic symptoms are present and more ominous signs—such as weight loss, anemia, choking, chest pain, and difficulty swallowing—are absent, doctors usually do not need to perform any diagnostic tests to confirm the diagnosis of GERD. Rather, the doctor will treat the patient's symptoms with either a prescription medication or an over-the-counter medication. If all the symptoms clear up on the medication, then the diagnosis is confirmed and investigative tests are not needed. As noted in Chapter 3, treating a presumed illness to find out whether the treatment takes care of the symptoms is called a *therapeutic trial;* this approach may also be referred to as *empiric* (or practical) *treatment.* In this case, treatment is based on the assumption that the diagnosis is likely to be GERD. If the treatment for GERD works, then the empiric trial was successful, and the doctor is usually satisfied that the symptoms were most likely caused by GERD. In Chapter 1, Dr. Johnson treated Joe empirically when Joe first came to him describing GERD symptoms.

Many, many people do not have these classic symptoms of GERD, however. Some people notice only hoarseness in their voice, while others begin coughing at night even though they don't have a cold. Some people don't have any symptoms until they develop complications such as a stricture, and some people have symptoms suggestive of other disorders that can be serious and that need to be treated completely differently from GERD. People with chest pain who have heart disease instead of GERD, or people with breathing problems who have asthma, an infection, or emphysema instead of GERD, must be diagnosed and treated appropriately. It is important not to assume that their symptoms are due to GERD.

If a person has classic symptoms of GERD but a therapeutic trial does not clear up the symptoms, or if a person has some of the less common symptoms of GERD, especially symptoms that may indicate a more serious illness, then the physician will almost certainly want to investigate the symptoms more thoroughly using one or more of the tests described in this chapter. Some of these tests (upper endoscopy, 24-hour pH probe, esophageal manometry) are *invasive*, meaning that they involve entering the body. Other tests, including x-ray studies such as a barium swallow or an upper gastrointestinal series, are non-invasive. Each test is designed to provide specific information, and a patient may need to have more than one test so that the doctor can gather all of the information necessary for appropriate diagnosis and treatment.

Tests are often performed to eliminate ("rule out") possible diagnoses. For example, in an older person with new-onset GERD-like symptoms and difficulty swallowing, an upper endoscopy (also known as an EGD) may be performed to rule out esophageal cancer rather than to diagnose GERD. Most physicians form a mental list of possible diagnoses after interviewing and examining the patient. This complete list of possible diagnoses that can account for a specific symptom or constellation of symptoms is called the *differential diagnosis.* As testing proceeds and laboratory results return and follow-up patient visits are made, the list becomes shorter and shorter, until the final diagnosis is clear. Diagnostic testing, then, is the process of narrowing down the differential diagnosis until only one choice—the correct diagnosis— remains and thus is confirmed as the cause.

When a physician decides to order one or more tests to help make or confirm a diagnosis, he or she must consider the cost of the test, the availability of the test, the duration of the test, the need for sedation, and of course, the risks and benefits of the test. Most important, the doctor needs to consider carefully whether the specific test will answer the questions that have been posed, and whether the results will lead to a change in the patient's treatment plan. Clearly, if the test is un-likely to provide useful information or to affect treatment, in most instances it makes little sense to perform it.

Note that while all of these tests can be performed during preg-nancy, most doctors avoid performing them on pregnant women ow-ing to concern over possible side effects to the developing fetus. Doctors do not routinely recommend EGD during pregnancy, and they perform EGD during the first trimester only in emergency situations (see Chapter 9).

Some terms: The *prescribing doctor* is usually a doctor who has examined you and taken your medical history and who has ordered the test you are about to undergo. The *radiologist* is a medical specialist who has special training in performing radiology (x-ray) tests and interpreting the results of those tests; if necessary, the radiologist can administer medications through an intravenous catheter (also called an *i.v.*). The *technician* is someone with specialized training in conducting medical tests who assists the physician. The *endoscopist* is a specially trained physician (usually a gastroenterologist) with additional specialized training in performing and interpreting procedures using an endoscope (a lighted fiberoptic tube used to visualize the stomach and esophagus).

Barium Swallow

In addition to testing for GERD, a barium swallow can be used as a rough estimate of the motility (the muscle contractions) in the esophagus. Sometimes called an *esophagram,* a barium swallow is an outpatient test, meaning that the patient is not admitted to a hospital for the test. A barium swallow can be performed in the radiology suite of a hospital or in a radiologist's office. The test is usually performed in the morning, and the patient is instructed not to eat or drink anything after midnight the night before the test. No sedation or intravenous catheter is needed.

As the test begins, the patient takes small sips of a thick radio-opaque liquid, and x-rays of the esophagus are taken as the patient slowly sips the liquid. (*Radio-opaque* means not easily penetrated by x-rays. Radio-opaque objects like contrast dye show up on x-ray films as bright white areas.) If the physician is concerned about the possibility of a stricture, or narrowing, of the esophagus, the radiologist may also ask the patient to swallow a barium sulfate pill, usually half an inch in diameter. This pill is easy to swallow and later dissolves in the intestinal tract. If the patient does have a stricture, this pill makes it possible to visualize the stricture and estimate how narrow the esophagus is. As an example, if a patient has developed a stricture in the lower esophagus that is only a quarter of an inch in diameter, then a barium tablet half an inch in diameter will temporarily "hang up" or "catch" at this narrowed area. The barium pill will slowly dissolve and coat the lower esophagus, and help the radiologist better characterize the degree of the stricture (length and extent of narrowing).

Barium and other radio-opaque materials are used in this test because they can easily be seen on the x-ray machine. The liquid is usually *barium sulfate,* a thin white liquid that tastes chalky. Barium is an inert substance (it does not react with other chemicals or medicines) and is nonallergenic. A radio-opaque liquid called *gastrograffin* is sometimes used in this test instead of barium. Gastrograffin comes in a variety of flavors but is more expensive than barium and is usually reserved for special situations, such as when there is a concern over a possible leak or perforation in the esophagus, in which case barium is dangerous to use.

The patient may be standing or seated and may be asked to change positions as the test progresses—to lie down on his or her back or stomach. These changes in position can help the radiologist identify a hiatal hernia or a paraesophageal hernia. During the barium swallow the x-rays are focused only on the throat and the esophagus; x-rays of the stomach or of the duodenum (upper small intestine) are not taken unless an ulcer or other problem in those areas is suspected.

After the test the patient is usually free to leave immediately. Over the next two to three days the patient needs to drink large quantities of fluids, to make sure all of the barium passes through the gastrointestinal tract easily. The stool is likely to be very light or even chalky in color for the next 48 to 72 hours as the barium passes through the GI tract. Although this can be startling to the patient if he or she has not been warned in advance, it is not harmful.

The barium swallow has a number of advantages compared with some of the other tests used to diagnose GERD. First, it is very safe. There are almost no risks other than exposure to a small amount of radiation from the x-rays. It is also fairly inexpensive (approximately $200) and very convenient, as it can be performed in almost any radiology suite. And results of the test are usually available within 24 to 48 hours.

The barium swallow has some limitations, however. The first is that it does not allow direct visualization of the lining of the esophagus. In people with GERD, the mucosa (lining) of the esophagus usually shows signs of inflammation or irritation. This finding is very difficult to demonstrate on a barium swallow. In addition, this is not a good test to determine whether the person suffers from acid reflux. Most radiologists can artificially induce an episode of reflux in any patient, so it is expected that reflux will occur during a barium swallow. This doesn't tell the medical team anything about what the patient is experiencing in day-to-day life, however. A third limitation is that if an abnormality is seen during the procedure, nothing further can be done during the test. If there is evidence of a stricture, an ulcer, or some other type of lesion, the patient will need to be referred for endoscopy so that biopsies can be taken. Finally, the barium swallow is designed to investigate only the esophagus, so evidence of a problem in the stomach or duodenum may be missed.

Upper Gastrointestinal Series

The only significant difference between a barium swallow and an upper gastrointestinal series is that in the upper GI series the radiologist takes x-rays for a longer time, to follow the contrast material (the barium or gastrograffin) as it passes through the esophagus and stomach and into the duodenum. The advantage of this test is that it allows investigation of a greater portion of the upper GI tract, so it is possible to diagnose multiple problems in this area. It is not uncommon, for example, for someone to have both acid reflux disease and an ulcer in the stomach or duodenum.

To obtain a better x-ray, the radiologist may introduce some gas into the patient's stomach to help distend (expand) it. This is usually done by having the patient swallow a "fizzy" tablet that produces carbon dioxide in the stomach. This is very safe, but it may make the patient feel a little bloated or gassy. Overall the test takes only a few minutes longer than the barium swallow. It is slightly more expensive (approximately $250), and the dose of radiation is slightly higher, because additional x-rays are taken.

Upper Endoscopy

Upper endoscopy—also called EGD, for esophagogastroduodenoscopy—is one of the tests most commonly used by gastroenterologists to help diagnose GERD and to treat many of its complications (see Chapter 8). It is usually performed as an outpatient procedure, although it is often used in diagnosing and treating hospitalized patients, as well. The test requires insertion of an intravenous catheter so that medications can be given directly into the vein. This allows the medications to work much more quickly, and it also allows for smaller doses to be given than would be required with oral medications.

Conscious sedation is used to make the patient feel relaxed, comfortable, and sleepy (see below). Conscious sedation is different from general anesthesia in that the patient continues to breathe spontaneously and there is no need for a breathing tube to be inserted into the throat or for the patient to be connected to a breathing machine. The patient is connected to a machine that monitors the pulse, the blood pressure, and the oxygen content of the blood. In most endoscopy centers the patient wears oxygen tubing (nasal prongs) as well, just in case he or she gets too sleepy and the oxygen content of the blood starts to drop.

The patient is instructed not to eat or drink for eight hours before the test, and to arrive one hour before the procedure, when he or she is evaluated by the nursing staff and by the doctor (the endoscopist) who will be performing the procedure. Once the intravenous catheter has been inserted, the patient is wheeled into the endoscopy suite, and medications are administered through the i.v. to relax the patient and make him or her sleepy.

At the same time, the tongue and back of the mouth are numbed using a topical anesthetic. The most common topical anesthetics contain benzocaine. Although they don't taste very good, they do an effective job of numbing the mouth and tongue and eliminating the normal gag reflex that everyone has when something touches the back of the mouth. If the patient has dentures, they will be removed just before the tongue and mouth are anesthetized. Finally, a plastic mouth guard called a *bite block* is placed in the mouth between the upper and lower teeth to protect the mouth, tongue, and teeth.

Once the patient is relaxed, a long, thin, flexible lighted tube called an *endoscope* is gently inserted into the mouth, slid over the tongue, and then passed into the esophagus and down into the stomach (see Figure 4.1 *[A]*). During the procedure a small amount of air is pumped into the stomach to make it expand so that it can be seen clearly. This occasionally causes some minor discomfort during the test, but it is not dangerous. The muscular connection (called the *pylorus*) between the stomach and duodenum is also carefully examined during this test, as is the duodenum.

During the procedure, small forceps can be inserted into the stomach through the endoscope, so that the doctor can remove tiny pieces of tissue to examine under the microscope later. This tissue-gathering procedure is called a *biopsy.* Many people are concerned about this procedure, but the removal of this small piece of tissue is painless and is not dangerous.

The entire procedure usually lasts between 20 and 30 minutes. At its conclusion the endoscopist removes any air that might have been pumped into the stomach and then withdraws the endoscope. The patient is then returned to the same-day surgery suite and is observed for one to two hours until he or she is fully awake. Most patients remember checking in for the test and the start of the test, but they remember very little of the test after that point. Patients who have had an EGD are allowed to go home with a family member or friend. They are not allowed to drive themselves home because the medications used can sometimes make them sleepy or slow down their reflexes even hours after the test has been performed. In addition, patients are instructed not to make any major business or financial decisions later in the day, as the medications may affect the ability to think and make critical judgments.

The time elapsed from first arriving in the same-day surgery center to discharge is generally three to four hours. The endoscope is usually in the stomach or esophagus for about 15 to 20 minutes. If biopsies are taken, the results are usually available within a week.

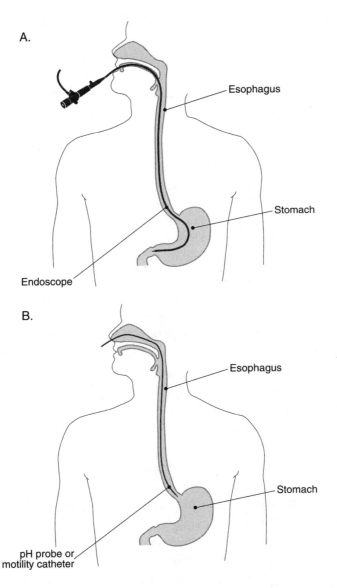

A.

Esophagus

Stomach

Endoscope

B.

Esophagus

Stomach

pH probe or
motility catheter

Figure 4.1. *(A)* A schematic of a patient undergoing an EGD, also called an upper endoscopy examination. The endoscope has been passed through the open mouth, over the tongue, down the esophagus, and into the stomach. *(B)* A schematic of a patient undergoing a motility study of the esophagus or a pH study. Here the catheter, which is thinner than the standard endoscope pictured in *(A)*, is passed through the nose and then down the esophagus.

Upper endoscopy has many positive attributes as a test to diagnose GERD. First, EGD allows direct inspection and visualization of the lining of the esophagus and stomach. If acid reflux has caused inflammation, scarring, or even an ulcer of the esophagus, these changes can easily be seen. Evidence of a stomach or duodenal ulcer can also be seen.

Second, if any abnormalities of the esophageal lining are noted, biopsies can be taken. As noted in Chapter 3, symptoms are a poor indication both of the actual amount of acid that is refluxed into the esophagus and of the extent of damage. The knowledge that their stomach and esophagus look normal, and that biopsies of the esophagus are normal, even when they have had severe symptoms, is very reassuring to most people.

Third, people with long-term acid reflux disease are at risk of developing Barrett's esophagus, a precancerous condition of the esophagus (see Chapter 8). Patients with longstanding GERD usually need to have biopsies taken from the lower end of the esophagus (the distal esophagus) to determine whether Barrett's has developed and, if Barrett's is present, to determine whether there is evidence of cancer.

Fourth, although invasive, EGD is generally safe. Most active endoscopy centers perform several thousand EGDs each year, and the risk of a complication is low.

EGD does have some limitations, the most obvious being that, unlike the barium swallow, it is invasive. Any invasive test (even inserting an i.v. into a small vein in the arm) has the potential for causing a complication. Potential complications of EGD include bleeding, infection (very rare), aspiration (inhaling stomach contents into the lungs), or a superficial tear in the esophagus or stomach. The worst potential complication is a *perforation*, which is a complete tear through the muscular wall of either the esophagus or stomach; this occurs in fewer than 1 in 10,000 procedures. A perforation almost always requires emergency surgical repair.

A second limitation of EGD is that sedation is usually required (see below for a discussion of the medications used in EGD). Use of sedatives can cause complications (discussed later in this chapter), but when sedatives are carefully administered in small doses and pulse, blood pressure, and oxygen content are monitored, complications are uncommon. Some people do not want any sedation, and EGDs are sometimes performed without sedation. Some patients who ask for the procedure to be performed without sedation are nervous about the use of sedatives or have had allergic or adverse reactions to such medications in the past; others have had problems with drug addiction in the past. In these situations, EGD can still be performed, but it requires special teamwork between the patient and doctor. The doctor will spend extra time numbing the mouth and the back of the throat, and will carefully discuss the entire procedure to help the patient remain relaxed. The doctor may have the patient practice special breathing techniques to induce a state of relaxation. The patient will need to concentrate on not gagging or choking during the procedure, and he or she will need to follow all directions carefully. If the patient is properly anesthetized with a topical agent to the mouth and tongue and is completely relaxed and in control, the EGD usually proceeds well without i.v. sedation. However, most patients find it difficult to remain relaxed and in control, and most endoscopists do not recommend EGD without sedation.

Other considerations are the cost of and time required for this procedure. An EGD may cost between $600 and $1,000, reflecting the invasive nature of the test, the need for monitoring, the need for more support staff, the specialized training of the endoscopist, fees paid to the hospital or endoscopy center, and the potential for complications. The test takes longer than a barium swallow, and patients are usually sleepy after the test, so recovery takes longer, as well.

EGD is an exemplary diagnostic test, but because it is invasive, many patients would prefer to avoid it and have a barium swallow instead. It's important to use the appropriate test for the situation, however. For example, an EGD is strongly recommended for anyone who is concerned that he or she might be developing Barrett's esophagus and who has had heartburn for more than five years, even if the heartburn symptoms are well controlled. In addition, anyone who is on medications for GERD and is still having symptoms probably needs to undergo EGD. EGD, not barium swallow, is the best test to directly inspect the mucosa (lining) of the esophagus and look for esophagitis,

Barrett's esophagus, or an ulcer or erosion. In addition, the doctor can perform a biopsy of the esophagus if he or she sees an area that does not look normal. The biopsy can confirm the diagnosis of Barrett's and also indicate whether there is evidence of early cancer. A barium swallow is a good, safe test to identify the presence of a stricture, or narrowing, of the esophagus, but it is not as effective as an EGD in evaluating the esophageal mucosa.

Twenty-Four-Hour pH Probe

Some people have occasional episodes of acid reflux that are very uncomfortable and worrisome, even though they last only a short time. However, these brief episodes, regardless of whether they clear up on their own or with the use of medications, usually do not cause significant damage to the esophagus that can be seen on EGD. For the large group of people who have significant acid reflux that produces symptoms not considered classic (change in voice, laryngitis, chronic cough), the EGD may be entirely normal. Nevertheless, these people do suffer from acid reflux disease, and the best diagnostic test for them is usually the 24-hour pH probe.

This is often a second- or third-line test, then, performed only after a barium swallow or EGD has shown the need for additional testing. A 24-hour pH probe is most often performed in people who have developed complications from GERD, in people whose diagnosis is still in doubt after an x-ray study or EGD, or in people who are considering surgery for severe GERD. This test is designed to measure how much acid is refluxing into the esophagus (the pH level of the esophagus) over a 24-hour period. It is an *ambulatory* test, which means that the patient goes about his or her daily activities of eating, working, and sleeping while the test is going on.

What is pH, and why is the pH of the esophagus measured? The pH is a measurement that indicates whether a solution is acidic or alkaline (basic). A pH of 7.0 is considered neutral (water is a good example). A number lower than 7.0 indicates that the solution is acidic (vinegar is an example), while numbers higher than 7.0 indicate a basic solution (such as milk). Gastric secretions are usually at a low pH, usually less than pH 4.0, owing to the presence of hydrochloric acid. When acid is refluxed back up into the esophagus, which is normally neutral in pH, the pH of the esophagus drops into the acidic range.

This test measures not only the number of episodes of acid reflux over a 24-hour period but also how long the esophagus is in an acidic state. Most endoscopy centers that perform this test use a pH monitor that allows the patient to press a button on the monitoring unit to record when symptoms of acid reflux occur. In this manner the physician can determine whether there is any relationship between the patient's symptoms and the episodes of acid reflux.

The only preparation for the test is to avoid eating or drinking for five to six hours beforehand. Depending on the circumstances, the physician may ask the patient to continue taking any medications he or she is currently taking for acid reflux, or the physician may ask the patient to stop taking these medications three to five days before the procedure. Placement of the pH probe is usually performed in the endoscopy suite or a same-day surgery center. This test is performed without sedation or the use of an i.v. It involves passing a small, thin, flexible tube (called a *catheter*) through one nostril into the back of the throat and then down into the esophagus (see Figure 4.1 *[B]*). Placement of the tube is an easy matter, and most people tolerate it very well. The back of the patient's throat may be numbed with a topical agent, but most people don't require any numbing medicine. Placement of the tube generally takes 5 to 10 minutes. The tube is then securely taped to the nose, and the recording unit is worn around the waist.

The patient returns to the endoscopy suite in 24 hours to have the tube removed. During this time the patient is encouraged to eat, drink, work, exercise, sleep, and perform all usual physical activities. The tube does not interfere with eating or drinking. Most people go to work and perform their usual activities, but some are self-conscious about wearing the monitor and take a day off from work. Results of the test are usually available in the week after the test is performed.

The 24-hour pH probe is a very safe and useful test. The tube is soft and flexible, and the complication rate from this test is almost zero. Moreover, i.v. medications are not needed. This test can provide additional information about patients with severe symptoms who may have a normal EGD. It can confirm the presence of severe reflux disease in people who do not have mucosal inflammation or in anyone with uncommon symptoms of GERD.

What are the limitations of this test? First, not all endoscopy centers perform it, so patients must often be referred to an academic institution or a teaching hospital for the test. In addition, this test is somewhat expensive, costing, on average, $300 to $400. Finally, some people object to the test because they find it uncomfortable or because they dislike the idea of wearing the recording device for 24 hours.

Esophageal Manometry

Esophageal manometry is a test specially designed to measure the *motility* (muscular activity) of the esophagus. As discussed in Chapters 1 and 2, acid reflux disease is not a disease of too much acid; rather, it is a disease of gastric acid in the wrong place. Symptoms of heartburn occur when gastric acid refluxes back up into the esophagus for longer periods of time than normal, or refluxes into the esophagus more frequently than normal. Motility disorders (disorders of muscle contraction) can affect the esophagus so that the muscles in the wall of the esophagus fail to contract normally. This allows acid that has previously washed up into the esophagus to remain there for too long. Esophageal manometry is used to determine if there is a problem with the muscles in the lower esophageal sphincter or with the muscles in the wall of the esophagus.

Like the 24-hour pH probe, esophageal manometry is not the first test a physician would use to diagnose GERD. For the evaluation of patients with acid reflux disease, a pH probe may be performed in people with severe GERD, in people who continue to have severe symptoms despite regular use of appropriate medications, in people who continue to have symptoms and who have a normal EGD, or in people who are considering surgery for GERD. Esophageal manometry is also similar to the 24-hour pH probe with regard to the amount of preparation required and the lack of sedation.

This test is performed as an outpatient procedure and does not require the use of sedatives or the placement of an i.v. The only preparation is to refrain from eating and drinking for five to six hours beforehand. The test cannot be performed immediately after a barium swallow or upper GI series, because the barium could clog the equipment. Patients need to stop taking certain medications in the 24 to 48 hours prior to the test, because medications such as calcium-channel blockers (verapamil, diltiazem, nifedipine), sedatives, theophylline, narcotics, nitrates, and metoclopramide can alter the results of the study. If for health reasons these medicines cannot be temporarily discontinued, note of that will be made by the technician or doctor performing the test.

An esophageal motility study begins by passing a thin, flexible tube through one nostril down into the esophagus and into the upper stomach (see Figure 4.1 [B]). Although many patients are nervous about this procedure, almost everyone tolerates it very well. The test starts with the technician lubricating the nostril with water-soluble lubricant, which may or may not contain a numbing medicine like lidocaine. The tube is then gently slid into the nostril until it reaches the back of the nose, where the throat begins. The patient is asked to place his chin on his chest to help the tube drop down into the esophagus, and is then asked to swallow a small amount of water to help move the tube down through the esophagus. The technician may then adjust the catheter to place it at the junction of the esophagus and the stomach.

The first recordings are then made. The catheter measures the resting muscular tone of the lower and upper esophageal sphincters and determines how well these sphincters relax. The catheter also reveals how well the esophagus contracts and whether those contractions are appropriately timed.

The test usually starts with the patient taking several swallows without any food or liquid in the mouth (dry swallows). The patient is then given some water and asked to swallow again (wet swallows). This process is repeated several times as the catheter is gently moved up and down within the esophagus. During the test the position of the catheter is adjusted to ensure that the activity of the lower esophageal sphincter, the upper esophageal sphincter, and the body of the esophagus is properly monitored. The test lasts 30 to 60 minutes. The catheter is then removed, and the patient is allowed to go home. Results are usually available within a week after the test is performed.

Overall, esophageal manometry is safe, as it does not require an i.v. or any medications. Most people tolerate the test well without any choking or gagging, although if the patient cannot tolerate having a tube placed through the nose, or if he or she has had previous nasal surgery, the tube may be inserted over the tongue and into the esophagus. This placement through the mouth can cause gagging.

Esophageal manometry is moderately expensive—about $450. Not all endoscopy centers perform the test, so if your physician decides that you need it, you may be referred to an academic medical center, a large teaching hospital, or a specialized gastrointestinal motility center.

Medications Used during Upper Endoscopy

Upper endoscopy, or EGD, is a routine procedure that is safely performed many thousands of times each year at endoscopy centers (sometimes called *ambulatory surgery centers*), community hospitals, and academic medical centers. A number of different medications may be used to make sure that the patient is as comfortable as possible during the procedure, and to help ensure that the test can be performed as safely as possible (by keeping the patient relaxed and still).

Some patients are concerned that the medications used during endoscopy will cause them to become addicted to drugs. But the medications used during endoscopy do not cause addiction, for a variety of reasons. First, addiction to almost any type of medicine or drug usually requires repeated doses or trials of the medicine; the medicines used in endoscopy are given to the patient only *once,* on the day of the procedure. Second, most of the medications used in the endoscopy suite have a very short lifespan in the body, so they are eliminated before the body gets used to their effects. We are not aware of a single patient who has ever become addicted to one of these medicines after having undergone an endoscopy, or even several endoscopies.

Most endoscopy centers now use conscious sedation as the sedation technique for EGD; as noted above, this approach to sedation eliminates the breathing tube and ventilator used in general anesthesia.

Conscious sedation uses medications designed to keep the patient relaxed, comfortable, and free of discomfort or pain but still able to breathe on his or her own and respond appropriately to instructions or any physical discomfort encountered.

Some of the medications used provide amnesia for the time actually spent in the procedure. This explains why many patients remember being taken into the endoscopy suite and then waking up after the procedure is over, but nothing in between. This type of amnesia, in which a small amount of memory is lost forward in time, after the medicines are given, is called *anterograde amnesia* (when past memories are lost, this memory loss is called *retrograde amnesia*). There are four general classes of medications used to achieve conscious sedation during endoscopy: sedatives, narcotics, topical anesthetics, and others.

Sedatives

Sedatives, also called *anxiolytics,* are used to reduce anxiety and to produce a calming effect. Many drugs in this category also have hypnotic properties, which means that they produce drowsiness and encourage sleep. These effects are due to the action of sedatives on the central nervous system (brain and spinal cord). Safe administration of these medications involves giving them very slowly, in small quantities, through the i.v., and monitoring the patient's pulse, blood pressure, and oxygen content of the blood. Initial effects of the medication may include a feeling of calm, warmth, and total relaxation.

These medications generally have a short half-life, which means that they are broken down quickly in the body and their effects wear off fairly rapidly. Potential side effects include respiratory depression or cardiovascular depression, which means that the person's breathing slows down too much, or the pulse or blood pressure drops too low. Should this occur, the patient is usually given supplemental oxygen and intravenous fluids; the sedative effects can usually be reversed with the use of a medication called *flumazenil.*

The two most commonly used sedatives are midazolam and diazepam. Midazolam (brand name Versed) dissolves easily in water and thus rarely causes any irritation to the veins. It often produces significant anterograde amnesia, which is comforting to many people. Diazepam (brand name Valium) can be administered through an i.v. as well, although it is less easily dissolved in water and thus can sometimes cause irritation to the vein where it is injected.

Although frequent use of sedatives may lower pressure in the lower esophageal sphincter and thus increase reflux, the small amounts given at the time of the endoscopy will not affect the test. Insertion of the endoscope causes reflux (temporarily holds the LES open) in any case, and even this does not affect the test results, since during the EGD the physician is interested not in reflux per se but in its consequences.

Narcotics

As a class of medications, the term *narcotics* usually refers to opioids, which are derived from opium. Opium comes from the seed pod of the poppy flower, specifically *Papaver somniferum.* Morphine was the first substance isolated from opium; this was achieved in 1803 by the German scientist Sertürner, who named the substance *morphine* after Morpheus, the Greek god of dreams. Narcotics are used to provide sedation and to provide *analgesia* (relief from pain). Because narcotics act on the central nervous system to produce their effects, large doses have the potential to cause respiratory depression. The two most commonly used narcotic agents in the endoscopy suite are meperidine (Demerol) and fentanyl (Sublimaze). Morphine is occasionally used in patients who are allergic to meperidine.

Topical Anesthetics

Topical anesthetics are used to numb the tongue and the back of the throat. They also prevent or minimize the gag reflex. Although most of them do not taste very good, they are generally well tolerated, and the effects usually wear off in 20 to 60 minutes. The most commonly used agents are benzocaine sprays (Hurricane or Cetacaine) and lidocaine spray (Xylocaine). Topical anesthetics come in a variety of forms (think of Bactine spray, for example, or the tubes of antibiotic ointment with analgesic agents in your medicine cabinet); for the EGD, topical anesthetics are administered as a spray down the throat.

Other

Other medications are occasionally used during upper endoscopy. They include *glucagon,* a medicine used to slow down smooth muscle contractions in the gastrointestinal tract. Excessive contractions sometimes make endoscopy difficult, so glucagon can be useful in performing this test. *Benadryl* is a favorite antihistamine that is very safe when used intravenously; it helps induce sleep and decrease anxiety. *Propofol* is a newer intravenous anesthetic that has the advantages of acting very quickly and then wearing off quickly. It also appears to produce less nausea than some of the narcotics listed above. One limitation is that most centers require that an anesthesiologist be present to administer the medication, which adds substantial cost to the procedure. Propofol is not used routinely. *Vistaril* (hydroxyzine) and *Phenergan* (promethazine) are antihistamines that cause some sedation and can also be used to prevent nausea and vomiting.

Understanding what causes symptoms and how a diagnosis is reached is all very well, but what most people want, of course, is relief from symptoms and protection from complications. In the next part of the book we explore the options for treating GERD. And, as we'll stress throughout the next few chapters, appropriately treating GERD is the best way to avoid complications.

Part III

TREATMENT:
THE FOUR-STEP
APPROACH

Chapter 5

Step 1
Lifestyle Modifications

Hannah, a 22-year-old student from England, is spending a study year abroad in the United States. She never had any health concerns before, but six months after she began her studies here, Hannah started to experience typical GERD symptoms: frequent bouts of burning in her chest along with regurgitation of sour-tasting material into her throat. After a long day of classes and studying, what Hannah needed most was a good night's sleep. But each night when she went to bed, the symptoms popped up and kept her awake. For a while she thought the symptoms would go away on their own, and she didn't think it was necessary to visit the student health clinic. She began to make a connection between her symptoms and certain kinds of foods, such as a favorite late-night snack of pepperoni pizza, but she didn't know anything about GERD and what could be done to prevent it.

Hannah eventually decided that these symptoms were too annoying to put up with, and she went see the doctor at the clinic on campus. The doctor told her that she probably had GERD, and told her how to modify her lifestyle. The doctor also gave her a prescription for an H_2-blocker, but, not being a fan of taking any sort of medicine, Hannah decided to focus on the lifestyle changes. She stopped eating in the late evening when she stayed up late studying, cut back on her coffee and diet colas, and put last semester's textbooks under the legs at the head of her bed.

Hannah was surprised and very pleased to find that her symptoms of nighttime heartburn and regurgitation disappeared entirely. And she has found out by experimenting that if she strays from the "rules," she usually has another attack of GERD.

While over-the-counter and prescription antacids and other medications for treating the symptoms of GERD are widely available and can be very effective, the cornerstone of treatment for any disease or disorder is *prevention*. It is far better to avoid having attacks of GERD symptoms than to use medications. Especially as we get older, we tend to need medications to control a variety of problems, such as high blood pressure, diabetes, and arthritis; if we can avoid adding GERD medications to the mix, that's all to the good. Also, as we saw with Joe in Chapter 1, it's sometimes necessary to take increasingly stronger medications to control the symptoms of GERD; preventing symptoms may make it possible to avoid this progression of over-the-counter and prescription drugs. Again, the medications are available, and they are effective, but minimizing the *need* for medications is preferable to taking them.

In some people with intermittent or mild symptoms, lifestyle changes may be the only therapy needed to control GERD. The purpose of this chapter, then, is to describe in detail how to prevent episodes of symptomatic GERD by modifying diet and behaviors. Some people are exquisitely sensitive to the dietary and lifestyle factors that bring on GERD symptoms, while other people are not susceptible to GERD symptoms no matter what they eat or do. Most people are somewhere in the middle. It is helpful to know what foods and activities are potential problems so that you can be aware of what factors in your own life may be causing your symptoms.

Many people find it frustrating to try to identify what's causing their GERD symptoms. What appears to cause symptoms one week may not cause symptoms the next week, while a food or activity that seemed safe will suddenly appear to bring on a severe attack. One of the reasons it can be difficult to learn exactly what precipitates GERD in any specific individual is that there are false precipitants and true precipitants. A *true precipitant* causes symptoms. A *false precipitant* is associated one or more times with an attack of symptoms but has not actually caused them.

There is a saying in medicine and epidemiology (the study of the population patterns of disease) that "association does not equal causation." An example would be the person who drinks a cup of decaffeinated coffee and within an hour has an attack of severe heartburn. It seems logical to blame the decaffeinated coffee, since that was the only thing the person consumed before the attack began. What *else* could have done it? In fact, any number of things could have done it, including a change in position, a tight belt, and a random reflux episode. The decaffeinated coffee is an innocent bystander, a false precipitant; it is associated sequentially with the heartburn (first coffee, then heartburn), but it did not cause the heartburn.

From long observation and studies of many people, we know that certain classes of foods (like caffeinated beverages) and certain activities (like smoking) decrease pressure in the lower esophageal sphincter and therefore are likely to precipitate attacks of GERD symptoms, at least more frequently than foods or activities that do not affect LES pressure (see box, page 72). We know they are true precipitants, so that if someone says that drinking cola causes her to have heartburn, we can be fairly certain that cola is indeed a factor in her GERD. Some people with GERD symptoms find that cola does *not* precipitate symptoms, however, or that cola is only occasionally a problem (perhaps only when it is consumed at night). This does not mean that cola is a false precipitant; it only means that cola is a precipitant in some people and not in others.

If a food or lifestyle factor is known through scientific studies to decrease LES pressure, and if an episode of GERD symptoms follows its ingestion or occurrence, we can be reasonably certain that the association is real, and is causative. If, on the other hand, you notice an association between a food or event and an episode of GERD symptoms, and the food or event is not a known precipitant based on our knowledge of what causes GERD, you should probably be suspicious of the association, and you might want to do a little testing on your

Lifestyle Modifications for Acid Reflux Disease

Make dietary modifications
  Avoid acidic foods (citrus/tomato products)
  Avoid fatty foods/greasy foods
  Avoid chocolate and licorice
  Avoid peppermint and spearmint
  Avoid caffeine (coffee, cola, tea)
  Smaller, more frequent meals
  Light evening meal
  Minimum of three to four hours between the end of the
     evening meal and bedtime
  No snacks after dinner

Avoid alcohol

Avoid cigarette smoking

Elevate head of bed six inches

*Minimize or avoid medications that irritate the lining of the
  esophagus and stomach (after consultation with your doctor)*
  Doxycycline
  Iron or potassium supplements
  Nonsteroidal anti-inflammatory drugs (for example, aspirin,
     ibuprofen, naproxen)
  Quinidine

*Minimize or avoid medications that lower LES pressure (after
  consultation with your doctor)*
  Anticholinergics
  Calcium-channel blockers (diltiazem, nifedipine, verapamil)
  Nitrates
  Prostaglandins
  Sedatives (benzodiazepines)
  Theophylline

own to assess how reliably your association holds. In other words, watch how frequently the association does *not* hold. We are much more likely to notice positive associations (specific food = GERD) than we are to notice times when the same food or event is *not* associated with an attack (specific food = no GERD). This is called a *reporting bias,* meaning that we tend selectively to notice and report bad things over neutral things. It's a good idea to keep this in mind when evaluating the associations you may note between your GERD symptoms and specific foods or situations.

Let's now turn to those factors that are known to be true precipitants of GERD. Nearly all of these factors are within your control:

* the timing of meals in relation to bedtime and body position
* the size of meals and the amount of fat in the diet
* specific foods that are irritants or that lower LES pressure
* obesity and pregnancy
* cigarette smoking
* tight clothing
* medicines that lower LES pressure or injure the lining of the esophagus

Meals, Bedtime, and Body Position

It has long been known that eating—and, especially, eating a large or fatty meal—shortly before lying down is a precipitant of GERD symptoms in susceptible individuals. In fact, even in people without noticeable GERD symptoms, eating a large meal before bedtime is sometimes associated with abdominal discomfort. At the least, their uncomfortable feeling of fullness is made worse when they lie down flat.

This situation is a simple matter of physics. When a person is standing or sitting, the esophagus is higher than the stomach, and the downward pull of gravity helps prevent acid reflux. But when a person is lying down, the esophagus and stomach are essentially on the same level. In this position, acid can roll back up into the esophagus very easily, somewhat like the ocean coming in at high tide. When we lie flat, the contents of a full stomach tend to flow upward toward the

LES, which, as we learned in Chapter 2, is not a perfect barrier, even in people without GERD. For people with GERD, lying down within three or four hours after eating may cause any remaining food and acid in the stomach to reflux into the esophagus—the stimulus for symptoms of GERD. Hannah, at the beginning of this chapter, made two mistakes: she lay down soon after eating, and she ate foods that can cause GERD symptoms because of their high fat content (pepperoni pizza) and their caffeine (cola and coffee).

It's important to remain upright for at least three hours after a meal, and longer after a large or heavy meal. Another step to take to avoid reflux episodes is to elevate the head of the bed. For many people with GERD, nighttime is the time when they develop symptoms. This is true in part because when we are asleep, we produce less saliva and swallow less often. Swallowing saliva helps neutralize and clear away any refluxed acid; less swallowing means that the stomach acid is more concentrated—stronger—and therefore more likely to cause irritation. While elevating the head of the bed does not increase the amount of saliva or the frequency of swallowing, it does help reduce the flow of stomach acid into the lower esophagus. Elevating the head of the bed can often markedly improve GERD symptoms.

Here's the trick: The most obvious approach to elevating the head— using two or more pillows—is usually ineffective, because pillows raise only the head and neck, not the chest, where most of the esophagus and the LES are located. The most effective way to elevate the esophagus and LES is to place something under the mattress, such as a bed wedge (shaped like an elongated pyramid turned on its side; these may be purchased in a department store or medical supply store) or an escalating series of telephone books (one at midback level, two stacked under the upper back, and three stacked under the head and neck). Bed blocks are another option. These are placed under the legs at the head of the bed to achieve a sloping elevation from foot to head. The most costly approach is a hospital-type bed with manual or electric position adjustments.

For some people who do not notice nighttime symptoms but who have other symptoms or complications, elevating the head of the bed by about six inches and avoiding eating for several hours before lying down are recommended steps to promote esophageal healing. These steps are recommended for people with documented esophagitis even if they have no symptoms at all.

Meal Size and Dietary Fat

It's just logical that large meals would precipitate GERD symptoms. The bigger the meal, the more acid the stomach secretes to help in digestion, and the more acid there is, the more likely it is that some of it will find its way past the barrier of the lower esophageal sphincter into the esophagus. Big meals also take somewhat longer for the stomach to process, increasing the duration of the acid secretion as well as the volume. Finally, large meals distend the stomach, which may increase the amount of time the lower esophageal sphincter is relaxed.

The amount of fat in a person's diet is also important, because large amounts of dietary fat lead to obesity (another risk factor for GERD, as described in more detail below) but also because dietary fat is a powerful relaxer of the LES and stimulates the production of stomach acid. Dietary fat is found in many snack foods and desserts as well as in meats, fried foods, rich sauces, cheeses, full-fat dairy products, nuts, cooking oils, salad dressings, and butter and related spreads and condiments. These foods are most commonly consumed at the evening meal. Choosing a diet with an emphasis on reduced-fat or fat-free versions of these foods, along with generous servings of whole grains, vegetables, and fruits, is a good way to lower the fat content of your diet. This approach to eating is beneficial not only for its GERD-improving properties but also for decreasing the risk of heart disease, obesity, and some forms of cancer.

Foods to Avoid

Many people know from experience that they will suffer from an episode of heartburn if they indulge in a late-evening meal full of rich, fatty foods accompanied by a glass of wine or two. This is a potent combination, because fatty foods cause the normal emptying of the stomach to be delayed, which allows acid (and possibly also bile) to linger too long in the stomach, and both alcohol and fatty foods cause the LES to relax. Both of these conditions—acid lingering in the stomach and a relaxed LES—make it more likely that acid will reflux into the esophagus.

Adopting a diet lower in fat is an important general health rule. In addition, there are several specific foods to avoid if you have GERD symptoms. These foods can cause problems in two ways. First, some foods lower LES pressure. Foods to avoid in this category are alcohol, caffeine, chocolate, licorice, peppermint, spearmint, and theophylline-containing teas. Certain foods should be avoided because they are natural irritants to the stomach and esophagus. These include (again) alcohol and caffeinated beverages (especially coffee), as well as highly acidic foods such as citrus and pineapple juices, onions, and tomato juice. Observe and experiment to find out which of these foods are safe for you and which of them cause problems.

Obesity and Pregnancy

Obesity is a risk factor for GERD both because of its physical effects on the body and because the type of diet that often leads to obesity is generally a diet high in fat content. Obesity, particularly when the person has a large waist circumference (abdominal obesity, sometimes called *apple-shaped*), increases the pressure inside the abdominal cavity, which includes the stomach. This, in turn, increases the workload on the lower esophageal sphincter, which is then less likely to be an effective barrier against reflux of stomach acid. As we have seen, a high-fat diet increases the risk of symptomatic GERD. Someone who is obese is more likely to eat foods that are high in fat and to eat larger but fewer meals per day. The strain on the LES combined with the dietary factors means that there is an increased risk of GERD in someone who is obese.

Many women develop heartburn during pregnancy. This occurs for two reasons. First, there is an increase in the pressure on the abdominal cavity as the fetus grows and the uterus enlarges. This pressure changes the anatomy of both the stomach and the gastroesophageal junction, and these physical changes make it easier for acid to reflux into the esophagus. Several studies have shown that LES pressure declines as pregnancy progresses, and this low pressure, too, increases the likelihood that reflux will occur. Second, levels of both estrogen and progesterone in the blood are elevated during pregnancy; elevated levels of both of these sex hormones cause the LES to relax (see Chapter 9).

Weight loss, through either dieting or (for a pregnant woman) delivery, usually improves or even eliminates GERD symptoms. Even modest amounts of weight loss in someone who is obese can lead to an improvement of symptoms right from the beginning, perhaps because the person is eating a lower-fat diet. A natural corollary to the effect of weight loss is the effect of weight gain: it can bring about GERD symptoms or make existing symptoms worse.

While we're on the subject of weight loss, we should note that exercise can increase intra-abdominal pressure, which in turn decreases the effectiveness of the lower esophageal sphincter (tight clothing can have the same effect; see below). Position changes during exercise may also precipitate reflux. These changes are reversed as soon as the exercise is finished, fortunately.

Nicotine

Cigarette smoking is a known risk factor for both GERD and ulcers of the stomach and duodenum (this is also true, though to a lesser extent, of cigar and pipe smoking). Smokers are also more likely to suffer from complications of GERD, such as esophagitis, Barrett's esophagus, and esophageal cancer (with or without GERD).

Nicotine appears to be a culprit in GERD because it lowers pressure in the lower esophageal sphincter. In addition, smoking may directly irritate the esophagus, and it may also cause irritation indirectly, because cigarette smoking may decrease production of saliva, which helps protect the esophagus from acid. This means that any acid reflux will be more likely to cause damage in smokers than in nonsmokers, and that existing acid damage will be less likely to heal.

Stopping smoking has an immediate beneficial effect on GERD symptoms and risks (as if we needed yet another reason to quit smoking). It can be very difficult to quit smoking and stay away from cigarettes, but a physician can prescribe medications or a nicotine patch to improve the chances of success. These aids are particularly effective when used in combination with techniques of behavior modification, which can be learned either individually or in classes run by health professionals.

Tight Clothing

Clothes that fit tightly around the waist are common culprits in increasing intra-abdominal pressure (and decreasing the effectiveness of the lower esophageal sphincter). Pants or a belt that fits just snugly when you are standing up may become downright tight and increase intra-abdominal pressure when you are seated or leaning forward or after you have eaten a meal. Elastic waistbands are sometimes a problem: although they stretch, they may put constant pressure on the abdomen, especially after a meal, when such pressure is least desirable. And, unlike belted clothes, an elastic waistband cannot be let out. Girdles and similar "control" garments are also likely to increase intra-abdominal pressure.

Medicines That Cause Symptoms of GERD

While most medicines are not a problem for people who suffer from GERD, there are two ways in which medicines can make GERD symptoms worse. First, some medicines, like some foods, can be irritants to the lining of the esophagus and stomach. These medications may damage mucosal tissues when an episode of acid reflux occurs, if the acid contains chemicals from these medications. Medicines in this category include nonsteroidal anti-inflammatory drugs (such as aspirin, ibuprofen, and naproxen), some antibiotics (such as doxycycline), iron pills, potassium supplements, and the heart medicine quinidine.

Second, some medicines reduce pressure in the lower esophageal sphincter, thus increasing the frequency and severity of acid reflux. Medicines of this kind include nitrates, used to treat angina; theophylline, used to treat asthma; and calcium-channel blockers, used in hypertension and heart disease. (See box, page 72, for a complete list.)

While an alternative medicine may be available that does not increase GERD symptoms (for example, acetaminophen as a substitute for aspirin or ibuprofen to control pain or fever), sometimes there are no appropriate substitutions. It's always important to consult your primary health care provider before making any changes in your medications or stopping a medication for any reason, including GERD. On the other hand, your care provider may not be aware of the effect of the medication on your GERD, and if you inform him or her, it is possible that changes can be made.

In this chapter we have reviewed the lifestyle and dietary factors that can be adjusted to decrease the risk of GERD as well as the frequency or severity of symptoms. These adjustments may be all you need to relieve your symptoms of GERD. If following these recommendations for lifestyle changes does not eliminate or at least dramatically improve your symptoms, however, it may be time to add some medications for increased relief. We begin the discussion of the treatment of GERD with medications in the next chapter.

Chapter 6

Step 2

Over-the-Counter Medicines

Most people who have GERD do not suffer symptoms every day, and their episodes of reflux are brief, lasting only a few minutes or a few hours. Also, many people can predict when they will have symptoms of GERD. Based on their previous experience, they know what factors precipitate GERD symptoms for them. Fortunately, most episodes of acid reflux that are brought on by overeating, eating the wrong foods, or lying down too soon after a meal can be brought under control with over-the-counter (OTC) medications, even if such episodes cannot be avoided altogether by the lifestyle changes described in the previous chapter.

Over-the-counter heartburn medications are clearly needed—they account for over $1 billion a year in sales in the United States alone. These medications also offer several advantages for people who occasionally suffer from GERD: They are widely available in pharmacies, drugstores, and large supermarkets that have pharmacies within them. They generally provide quick relief. They are fairly inexpensive, especially when compared with prescription medications. They are easy to take, and most of them taste reasonably pleasant. All of them are convenient to use and can be taken without any special preparation. They can be carried in a pocket, purse, or backpack, so they are available when needed. They are very safe when used properly, and side effects are exceedingly uncommon. Finally, they rarely interact with any prescription medications that are being taken at the same time.

When lifestyle changes and nonprescription medications don't control symptoms, then a doctor can prescribe stronger and different medications. These medications are taken daily or twice daily and are very safe. With any medication used on a daily basis, however, there is always the potential for side effects or for an unpleasant or even dangerous drug interaction to occur with another medication being taken at the same time. (In Chapter 7 we discuss prescription medications for treating GERD.)

In this chapter we describe the various types of OTC medications as well as home remedies that can be used to treat GERD when symptoms occur infrequently and are not associated with any warning signs, such as chest pain, difficulty swallowing, choking, unintentional weight loss, low blood count, or evidence of bleeding. OTC medicines used to treat intermittent heartburn can be divided into four general categories: topical agents, which coat the lining of the esophagus and stomach; antacids; H_2-blockers; and home remedies.

Before we describe specific agents, it's important to set out some general guidelines in using these agents. For example, *OTC medicines should be used only occasionally, and only for brief periods of time.* If you need to take 10 Tums or Rolaids tablets each day, every day of the week, then even if these medications control your symptoms, you need to be taking a stronger medicine, and *you should see your doctor.* In addition, if you use these medicines regularly for longer than two weeks, or if you experience warning signs, then you need to see your doctor.

Women who are pregnant or breastfeeding should consult their physician before taking *any* medications, whether over-the-counter or prescription. Many women prefer to avoid all medications during pregnancy other than the vitamins and minerals prescribed by their doctor. They will put up with the symptoms of heartburn, knowing that when the baby is born the symptoms will almost always disappear. If the symptoms are too severe to live with, then any of the antacids described in this chapter can be used on an as-needed basis, with a doctor's approval. Some women find that two to three teaspoons of an antacid suspension (Maalox or Mylanta II) before bedtime is all they need to prevent nightly heartburn. If symptoms persist despite chronic antacid use, prescription medications may be needed. (Chapter 9 discusses GERD in pregnancy in more detail.)

Also, even though side effects are uncommon with these agents, *all medications have the potential to cause side effects.* Potential side effects of each of the specific OTC medications and home remedies are discussed in this chapter. Generally speaking, however, we can say that any medication that contains *magnesium* has the potential to cause diarrhea. Medications containing magnesium should also be used very cautiously by a person with poor kidney function *(renal insufficiency),* because magnesium can accumulate in the body to high levels if the kidneys are unable to dispose of it properly. Also, any agent that contains *aluminum* has the potential to act as a constipating agent and, if used routinely, to lower levels of phosphate in the blood, which can cause bone weakening *(osteomalacia).* Finally, agents that contain *calcium* have the (uncommon) potential to cause kidney stones and may lead to elevated calcium levels in the blood.

It is important to note that many of the over-the-counter medicines described here contain *sodium,* a component of salt (which is *sodium chloride*). If you are on a salt-restricted diet, you will need to read labels carefully to make sure you do not ingest too much sodium. Any person with occasional episodes of heartburn who has chronic kidney problems, renal insufficiency, or a history of congestive heart failure should talk with his or her doctor about the benefits and risks of the various OTC medicines. Antacids that can safely be used on an occasional basis by people with heart failure are those that are low in salt, such as Gelusil, Mylanta DS, Nephrox suspension, Rolaids, and Titralac. Di-Gel is sodium-free. Nephrox does not contain magnesium and thus is safe for occasional use by someone with poor kidney function. (Box on page 83 indicates which OTC antacids contain no sodium or are low in sodium and which are sugar-free or lactose- and galactose-free.)

We have heard about people who occasionally drink a whole bottle of Maalox in one day. Although drinking 10 or 12 ounces of Maalox at

Common Acid Reflux Medications Available without a Prescription

Medications containing aluminum

AlternaGEL

Amphojel

Gaviscon

Nephrox

Medications containing magnesium

Di-Gel

Phillips' Milk of Magnesia

Rolaids

Medications containing both aluminum and magnesium

Gelusil

Maalox

Mylanta

Lactose- and galactose-free medications

Axid AR

Maalox

Mylanta

Riopan

Rolaids

Tums

Zantac 75

Sodium-free medications

Di-Gel

Low-sodium medications

Gelusil

Maalox HRF

Mylanta DS

Nephrox suspension

Rolaids

Titralac

Sugar-free medications

Amphojel suspension

Amphojel tablets

Di-Gel liquid

Gaviscon liquid

Nephrox suspension

Riopan suspension

Tagamet HB

Titralac

Zantac 75

H$_2$-blockers

Axid AR (nizatidine)

Pepcid AC, Mylanta AR
(famotidine)

Tagamet HB (cimetidine)

Zantac 75 (ranitidine)

one time is probably not dangerous for a young person who does not have heart or kidney problems, it is not recommended and clearly is not safe to do repeatedly. More important, what this tells us is that such a person most likely has severe heartburn and should be on a stronger medicine to control symptoms. If heartburn is not well controlled, it may be causing permanent damage to the person's esophagus. *Anyone who feels the need to take a great deal of an OTC medication needs to see a doctor for appropriate treatment of severe heartburn.*

Another important warning applies to anyone taking the antibiotic tetracycline. *Tetracycline and antacids should not be taken at the same time.* Any antacid that contains aluminum, magnesium, or calcium can bind to tetracycline and decrease the amount of antibiotic that is absorbed, potentially making the antibiotic less effective. Plan on taking the antacid one to two hours before, or after, the dose of tetracycline.

Before beginning our discussion of specific medications, we should also note that the approximate cost per day of the medications given here should be used only as a guide in choosing the most appropriate medication. The cost listed here is based on an *average* daily dose of the medication, not on the *maximum* dose that can be used each day. We surveyed three different pharmacies in the Washington-Baltimore area to get an idea of the price of these medications. We used non-sale prices, and we based the average cost on the purchase of a large amount of the medication—that is, we used the regular cost of a package of 100 tablets or a pint bottle (16 ounces) of liquid medication, rather than the cost of a small packet of tablets (generally 8 or 10) or a one-day dose of liquid medication (generally 2 ounces). Your cost may be much different, depending on where you live, the amount of medication you buy, and the amount of competition in your area between pharmacies.

Topical Agents

Gaviscon (alginic acid). Alginic acid is a topical agent designed to mix with the mucus and saliva in the esophagus and stomach to form a "pool" of liquid that floats on top of the mucosal lining of these two organs. This pool acts as a barrier to protect the cells and tissues beneath the mucosal lining from the caustic actions of acid. Alginic acid is sold under the brand name Gaviscon in both liquid and tablet form. It is generally thought to work better during the day than at night.

The active ingredients of Gaviscon are aluminum hydroxide and magnesium trisilicate. Two to 4 tablets can be taken up to 4 times a day if necessary. The maximum dose is 16 tablets in 24 hours. One to 2 tablespoons of Gaviscon regular-strength liquid can be taken up to 4 times a day, with a maximum dose of 8 tablespoons in 24 hours. Gaviscon should not be taken at the same time as the antibiotic tetracycline because it may prevent full absorption of the antibiotic. People on a salt-restricted diet should use this agent carefully. *Onset of action:* minutes. *Duration of action:* hours. *Approximate cost per day:* less than $1.00.

Carafate (sucralfate). Sucralfate (aluminum sucrose sulfate) is a coating agent available only by prescription, but it is mentioned here because it acts somewhat like a topical agent. It acts by coating the lining of the esophagus and stomach and protecting them from the harmful effects of stomach acid. Sucralfate (brand name Carafate) may provide additional benefits by increasing the rate of healing of the esophagus if it has already been damaged by stomach acid. One tablet of sucralfate is mixed with water until it forms a *slurry* (or suspension); this is taken 4 times a day to coat the esophagus effectively. There are no significant side effects, although some people believe that this medication makes them constipated. *Onset of action:* minutes to hours. *Duration of action:* hours. *Approximate cost per day:* $4.00.

Antacids

Antacids are useful in treating GERD because they are weak bases (their pH is greater than 7.0) and therefore convert the caustic and potentially dangerous hydrochloric acid found in stomach acid into neutral water and a salt. Antacids also decrease the potential caustic effect of pepsin, another chemical found in gastric secretions. As discussed in Chapter 2, pepsin is a digestive enzyme that helps break down the proteins found in food. It may also play a role in the development of heartburn. Pepsin is active, or able to work, only in acidic conditions. When the pH of the esophagus is greater than 4.0 or 5.0, pepsin will not injure the esophageal lining. These are the two major actions of antacids: neutralizing stomach acid and preventing pepsin from working.

The amount of medicine needed to relieve symptoms of heartburn and regurgitation varies from person to person, based on a number of different variables. These variables include body size, weight, use of other medications, severity of symptoms, amount of acid that needs to be neutralized, and size and time of last meal. The form of the antacid used—solid tablets or liquid—may affect response to treatment, as well. One small study showed that chewable antacids provide more protection from acid reflux than the same medication taken in liquid form, though liquids generally act faster.

Listed below, in alphabetical order by brand name (also called trade name), are antacids that can be bought at most pharmacies, drug stores, and larger grocery stores. The active ingredients are given in parentheses after each trade name. The recommended dose, common side effects, onset and duration of action, and cost are also noted. Whenever using OTC or prescription medications, read the label carefully before taking any of the medication.

Alka-Seltzer (sodium bicarbonate). Two tablets every 4 hours, with a maximum dose of 8 tablets in 24 hours. Patients on a salt-restricted diet should use this medication carefully. Alka-Seltzer is listed here for the sake of completeness because it is so widely used. We usually do *not* recommend it for heartburn pain, however, because it also contains aspirin and citric acid, both of which can further irritate an already inflamed and irritated esophagus. Chronic use can cause ringing of the ears *(tinnitus)* due to the aspirin, and the aspirin can also cause stomach upset or even an ulcer. *Onset of action:* minutes. *Duration of action:* hours. *Approximate cost per day:* less than $1.00.

AlternaGEL (aluminum hydroxide). One to 2 teaspoons 4 times a day if necessary, with a maximum dose of 8 teaspoons in 24 hours. Chronic use can lead to depletion of phosphorus from the body and may weaken the bones in people with kidney failure who are on dialysis. Like other aluminum-containing drugs, it may cause constipation. AlternaGEL should not be taken at the same time as the antibiotic tetracycline because it may prevent full absorption of the antibiotic. *Onset of action:* minutes. *Duration of action:* hours. *Approximate cost per day:* $1.00.

Amphojel (aluminum hydroxide). Two teaspoons (10 mls) 5 or 6 times a day, or 1 to 2 tablets (0.6 g) every 4 to 6 hours. The maximum dose is 12 teaspoons in 24 hours, or 6 tablets in 24 hours. Patients with kidney failure who are on dialysis need to be careful if they use this medication on a chronic basis because it may worsen thinning of the bones *(osteomalacia)*. Like other aluminum-containing drugs, it may cause constipation. Amphojel should not be taken at the same time as the antibiotic tetracycline because it may prevent full absorption of the antibiotic. *Onset of action:* minutes. *Duration of action:* hours. *Approximate cost per day:* $1.50.

Di-Gel (calcium carbonate, magnesium hydroxide, simethicone). Two to 4 teaspoons every 2 hours as necessary, with a maximum dose of 20 teaspoons in 24 hours, or 1 to 2 tablets every 2 hours, with a maximum dose of 24 tablets in 24 hours. Di-Gel is sodium-free and therefore generally safe for someone on a sodium-restricted diet. It should not be taken at the same time as the antibiotic tetracycline because it may prevent full absorption of the antibiotic. Simethicone is designed to break up bubbles of gas in the stomach, which may reduce abdominal discomfort. *Onset of action:* minutes. *Duration of action:* hours. *Approximate cost per day:* less than $1.00.

Gelusil (aluminum hydroxide, magnesium hydroxide, simethicone). One to 2 teaspoons every 4 to 6 hours, or 2 to 4 tablets every 4 to 6 hours. Maximum dose is 12 teaspoons in 24 hours, or 12 tablets in 24 hours. Sodium-free and sugar-free. Gelusil should not be taken at the same time as the antibiotic tetracycline because it may prevent full absorption of the antibiotic. *Onset of action:* minutes. *Duration of action:* hours. *Approximate cost per day:* less than $1.00.

Maalox and Extra Strength Maalox (aluminum hydroxide, magnesium hydroxide). For regular Maalox, 2 to 4 teaspoons can be taken up to 4 times a day. Maximum dose should not exceed 16 teaspoons in 24 hours. The aluminum and magnesium help to balance each other out, and therefore problems with either constipation or diarrhea are uncommon. People with poor kidney function should use this agent carefully, because the magnesium can accumulate in the body to high levels. Extra Strength Maalox contains simethicone, which can help break up larger gas bubbles into smaller gas bubbles. The recommended dose of Extra Strength Maalox is 2 to 4 teaspoons 4 times a day if needed. Maalox and Extra Strength Maalox should not be taken at the same time as the antibiotic tetracycline because it may prevent full absorption of the antibiotic. *Onset of action:* minutes. *Duration of action:* hours. *Approximate cost per day:* less than $1.00.

Mylanta (aluminum hydroxide, magnesium hydroxide, simethicone). Two to 4 teaspoons or 2 to 4 gelatin capsules (gelcaps) up to 4 times a day if necessary. Maximum dose is 12 capsules in 24 hours, or 24 teaspoons in 24 hours. The aluminum and magnesium help to balance each other out, and therefore problems with either constipation or diarrhea are uncommon. People with poor kidney function should use this agent carefully, because the magnesium can accumulate in the body to high levels. Mylanta should not be taken at the same time as the antibiotic tetracycline because it may prevent full absorption of the antibiotic. *Onset of action:* minutes. *Duration of action:* hours. *Approximate cost per day:* less than $1.00.

Mylanta DS (aluminum hydroxide, magnesium hydroxide, simethicone). This is the same medicine as Mylanta, with the quantities of all the active ingredients doubled. (See above for cautions.) Two to 4 teaspoons up to 4 times a day, with a maximum dose of 12 teaspoons in 24 hours. *Onset of action:* minutes. *Duration of action:* hours. *Approximate cost per day:* less than $1.00.

Nephrox suspension (aluminum hydroxide). Two teaspoons up to 4 times a day if necessary, with a maximum dose of 8 teaspoons in 24 hours. This medication can be used in patients with poor kidney function because it does not contain magnesium and because it is low in sodium (19 mg/ounce). All the same, it should not be used on a chronic basis by anyone with poor kidney function or heart failure, or by anyone on a salt-restricted diet. Nephrox suspension should not be taken at the same time as the antibiotic tetracycline because it may prevent full absorption of the antibiotic. *Onset of action:* minutes. *Duration of action:* hours. *Approximate cost per day:* $1.25.

Phillips' Milk of Magnesia (magnesium hydroxide). One to 3 teaspoons up to 4 times a day, with a maximum dose of 12 teaspoons in 24 hours. (Higher doses are usually taken by people using the magnesium as a laxative to relieve constipation.) Patients with poor kidney function should use this medication carefully, because chronic use can lead to elevated magnesium levels in the blood. Phillips' Milk of Magnesia should not be taken at the same time as the antibiotic tetracycline because it may prevent full absorption of the antibiotic. *Onset of action:* minutes. *Duration of action:* hours. *Approximate cost per day:* less than $1.00.

Prelief (calcium glycerophosphate). This medication is very different from the others listed in this section. For one thing, it is classified as a dietary supplement, not as a drug. It is supplied as either tablets or a packet of granules that are designed to be mixed with acidic food before eating the food. The calcium glycerophosphate neutralizes the acid in the food and thus minimizes stomach upset and potentially decreases symptoms of acid reflux. For example, 1 or 2 tablets or packets should neutralize most of the acid contained in a single aspirin or ibuprofen tablet. To help neutralize acid, the packets can safely be mixed with foods or drinks such as tomato-based sauces, citrus drinks, coffee, tea, wine, beer, and cola drinks. The manufacturers do not specify a daily maximum dose. Chronic use may lead to elevated and potentially dangerous blood calcium levels, however, so we urge caution. Prelief should not be taken at the same time as the antibiotic tetracycline because it may prevent full absorption of the antibiotic. *Onset of action:* minutes. *Duration of action:* minutes to hours. *Approximate cost per day:* less than $1.00.

Riopan (magaldrate). One to 2 teaspoons up to 4 times a day, with a maximum dose of 8 teaspoons in 24 hours. People with poor kidney function should not use this medication chronically. Riopan should not be taken at the same time as the antibiotic tetracycline because it may prevent full absorption of the antibiotic. *Onset of action:* minutes. *Duration of action:* hours. *Approximate cost per day:* less than $1.00.

Rolaids (calcium carbonate, magnesium hydroxide). One to 4 tablets hourly as symptoms occur, with a maximum of 12 tablets in 24 hours. Low in sodium and thus safe for people on a sodium-restricted diet. Each tablet has 22 percent of the daily recommended intake of calcium. Rolaids should not be taken at the same time as the antibiotic tetracycline because it may prevent full absorption of the antibiotic. *Onset of action:* minutes. *Duration of action:* hours. *Approximate cost per day:* less than $1.00.

Titralac and Titralac Extra Strength (calcium carbonate). Two tablets every 2 to 3 hours as needed for Titralac, with a maximum dose of 19 tablets in 24 hours. One to 2 tablets every 2 to 3 hours for Titralac Extra Strength, with a maximum dose of 10 tablets in 24 hours. Titralac is very low in sodium (1.1 mg/tablet), which is important to those on a low-sodium diet. Titralac and Titralac Extra Strength should not be taken at the same time as the antibiotic tetracycline because it may prevent full absorption of the antibiotic. *Onset of action:* minutes. *Duration of action:* hours. *Approximate cost per day:* less than $1.00.

Tums (calcium carbonate). Two to 4 tablets up to 4 times a day if necessary, with a maximum dose of 16 tablets in 24 hours. Chronic use can cause constipation in addition to high calcium levels in the blood. High-dose chronic use may cause kidney stones. Tums should not be taken at the same time as the antibiotic tetracycline because it may prevent full absorption of the antibiotic. This medication is used by many people on a daily basis, even if they don't have heartburn, to help maintain calcium levels in bone and blood and thus reduce the risk of osteoporosis. *Onset of action:* minutes. *Duration of action:* hours. *Approximate cost per day:* less than $1.00.

H_2-Blockers

Nizatidine, cimetidine, famotidine, and ranitidine are the four types of H_2- (histamine type 2) blockers, all of which reduce acid secretion by inhibiting H_2 receptors on acid-secreting cells in the stomach. All of the H_2-blockers sold without prescription are at a lower dose than is available by prescription. In our opinion, the four drugs are all very similar with regard to their ability to neutralize acid, as long as comparable doses are used: 75 mg of nizatidine is considered equal to 200 mg of cimetidine, which equals 10 mg of famotidine, which equals 75 mg of ranitidine. Women who are pregnant or breastfeeding should discuss the use of H_2-blockers with their doctor. Side effects vary from

H_2-blocker to H_2-blocker (see Chapter 7 for more detail), and it's important to read the warning label carefully.

Many people find that certain types of food invariably produce heartburn. Common offenders include Mexican food, Italian food, and French food. Symptoms often occur because of the high fat content of the food, the way the food is prepared (frying), or the rich sauce that accompanies the food. Sometimes it is not just the food but the fact that the meal is larger than usual, or is eaten later in the evening than usual, or is accompanied by alcohol or caffeine. Over-the-counter antacids are often effective in treating symptoms once they occur. But if there is a food or type of meal that reliably produces an episode of heartburn for you, you might want to take one of the OTC H_2-blockers one hour *before* you eat that food. These agents are safe, reasonably inexpensive, and generally effective in preventing episodes of heartburn if taken before eating.

Axid AR (nizatidine). Nizatidine is an H_2-blocker that inhibits H_2 receptors and reduces secretion of stomach acid. The usual dose is 1 tablet (75 mg) every 12 hours, with a maximum dose of 2 tablets in 24 hours. Women who are pregnant or breastfeeding should talk with their doctor before taking this medication. *Onset of action:* less than 1 hour. *Duration of action:* hours. *Approximate cost per day:* less than $1.00.

Mylanta AR Acid Reducer (famotidine). Although its name makes it sound like just one more variation of the original Mylanta formula, this medication is very different. The active ingredient is famotidine, another H_2-blocker that reduces secretion of stomach acid. It was originally available only as a prescription in a 20-mg dose, but now it can be purchased OTC at a lower dose (10-mg tablets). In OTC strength, 1 tablet (10 mg) can be taken twice daily. Many people use this medicine prophylactically (to prevent heartburn from occurring), in which case 1 tablet is taken 1 to 2 hours before eating a meal that may cause heartburn. Women who are pregnant or breastfeeding should talk with their doctor before taking this medication. Maximum dose is 2 tablets in 24 hours. *Onset of action:* less than 1 hour. *Duration of action:* hours. *Approximate cost per day:* less than $1.00.

Pepcid AC Acid Controller (famotidine). Famotidine is an H_2-blocker that inhibits H_2 receptors and reduces secretion of stomach acid. One tablet (10 mg) every 12 hours, with a maximum dose of 2 tablets in 24 hours. The active ingredient, famotidine, is the same active ingredient that is in Mylanta AR Acid Reliever. This medication should not be used for longer than 2 weeks; if you need it longer than that, then you should see your doctor, because the heartburn may be more severe than you suspect, or the discomfort may be due to something other than GERD. Women who are pregnant or breastfeeding should talk with their doctor before taking this medication. *Onset of action:* less than 1 hour. *Duration of action:* hours. *Approximate cost per day:* less than $1.00.

Tagamet HB 200 (cimetidine). Cimetidine is an H_2-blocker that inhibits H_2 receptors and reduces secretion of stomach acid. One tablet (200 mg) can be taken twice in 24 hours, usually 30 to 60 minutes before eating a meal that might cause heartburn. Potential interactions with other medications, such as warfarin (Coumadin, a blood thinner), theophylline (for chronic breathing problems like asthma), and phenytoin (seizure medicine), are more common than with antacids. Women who are pregnant or breastfeeding should talk with their doctor before taking this medication. *Onset of action:* approximately 1 hour. *Duration of action:* hours. *Approximate cost per day:* less than $1.00.

Zantac 75 (ranitidine). Ranitidine is an H_2-blocker that inhibits H_2 receptors and reduces secretion of stomach acid. Each tablet contains 75 mg of ranitidine, half the prescription dose of 150 mg. Up to 2 tablets can be taken in 24 hours. Many people take this medication 1 to 2 hours before eating a meal that they believe may cause heartburn. Women who are pregnant or breastfeeding should talk with their doctor before taking this medication. *Onset of action:* less than 1 hour. *Duration of action:* hours. *Approximate cost per day:* less than $1.00.

Home Remedies

Home remedies can be fun, convenient, low-cost, and effective—or not. The main thing to keep in mind with home remedies is that they should not be used as a substitute for seeking medical attention, especially if symptoms are severe or persist.

Baking soda (sodium bicarbonate). This time-proven home remedy has been used for over 80 years. When mixed with water, it is very effective in relieving heartburn and neutralizing stomach acid. One-half teaspoon in 4 ounces of water can be taken up to every 2 hours if necessary. The powder should be completely dissolved in water before drinking. Do not take more than 4 teaspoons (8 doses) over a 24-hour period. Baking soda is fast, safe, inexpensive, and reliable, but it contains sodium and can cause fluid retention in people with poor kidney function or heart failure. If used in large doses, it can make the blood too alkaline, which can be dangerous. It should not be used by pregnant women, because of the risk of fluid retention.

Bread. Many people think that white bread is a good antidote for acid reflux. The theory is that it "soaks up" the extra acid and prevents it from causing damage. Although it is an interesting idea, we don't think it works.

Buttermilk or milk. Milk is a popular remedy for heartburn among some people in farming communities in the Midwest and New England. The idea is that the milk will coat the stomach and esophagus to protect them from the acid, and that it will also help neutralize the acid. Cool, creamy milk may feel good going down, but its high fat content may lower pressure in the lower esophageal sphincter and actually make acid reflux *worse.*

Ice cream. The concept here is similar to that of milk: something cool and creamy to coat the esophagus and stomach. Some people may use the supposed "healing property" of ice cream as an excuse to indulge in a forbidden treat. Once again, the high fat content of the ice cream may relax the lower esophageal sphincter and actually make heartburn *worse.*

Conclusion and Recommendations

Occasional episodes of acid reflux can generally be safely treated with lifestyle modifications and an over-the-counter antacid. A large selection of reasonably priced medications are available without prescription.

Which of them do we recommend for people who suffer from occasional episodes of heartburn? We usually recommend the liquid form of either Mylanta DS or Extra Strength Maalox for those once-a-month episodes of heartburn associated with a large meal, a rich meal, or a late-night snack. Both of these products are good first choices because they begin to work quickly (rapid onset of action), they contain simethicone to help break up gas bubbles in the stomach, and they are easy to adjust to an effective dose by taking either a little more or a little less of the liquid. In addition, most people find them palatable.

For people who don't like taking liquid antacids or find them to be messy, the gelatin capsule form of Mylanta is effective, as are chewable Tums and Rolaids. These latter choices are more convenient as well, since it is easier to carry a few gelcaps or tablets in your pocket or purse then to carry around a bottle of liquid.

If the combination of lifestyle modifications and either liquid or chewable over-the-counter antacids does not solve the problem, then over-the-counter H_2-blockers are usually the next step. People who can predict when they are going to develop heartburn can take a single OTC H_2-blocker one hour before the meal. They may want to take a second dose before going to bed, to prevent nocturnal reflux. If this regimen does not work, then the next step is a visit to your doctor, first, to make sure that the problem really is acid reflux disease, and, second, to discuss the use of more potent medications.

We must emphasize that all of these OTC medications are designed for infrequent, intermittent use. If your symptoms seem typical of GERD and if they are relieved by a standard dose of one of the medications described above, then it is safe to take the OTC medications. If you think you have GERD, however, and if your symptoms *aren't* relieved by the maximum recommended dose of medication, then it is possible that your symptoms are due not to acid reflux but to some other problem, and you should see your doctor. We commonly see patients who have treated themselves for months or even years for "heartburn" and who actually had a chronic problem of the heart, lungs, gallbladder, stomach, liver, or even pancreas. If you find that you need to take OTC medications constantly or chronically (longer than two weeks), then, even if they work and relieve all of your symptoms, you should still see your doctor, because you may need to be on a stronger medication, or you may have another problem besides GERD.

Of the many medications available for treating the symptoms of GERD, this chapter has considered only the over-the-counter, or nonprescription, drugs. In the next chapter we turn to prescription medications—which include stronger versions of the OTC drugs as well as entirely different agents—and also to the surgical options for treating GERD.

Chapter 7

Steps 3 & 4

Prescription Medicines and Surgery

James, a 53-year-old accountant, thrived on long days at the office fueled by cigarettes and coffee. On some weekends he drank a fair amount of alcohol. James was having quite a bit of discomfort from classic GERD symptoms. His doctor advised him to change the habits that were contributing to his GERD symptoms, but James had not been able to quit smoking or cut back on coffee and cocktails. After a few months the doctor started him on Tagamet HB 200, a nonprescription H_2-blocker.

Eight weeks later James told his doctor that he was still having problems with heartburn and admitted that he hadn't been able to adhere to the lifestyle changes recommended to him. With this information, his doctor switched him to the prescription drug Prevacid, a once-a-day proton-pump inhibitor that did the trick for James's symptoms. But the doctor was slightly concerned that James's symptoms had not initially responded as well as he had hoped they would. In addition, James was over age 50 and had had heartburn symptoms for several years. For these reasons, the doctor referred James to a gastroenterologist, who performed an upper endoscopy.

During the EGD, the gastroenterologist saw mild esophagitis in James's lower esophagus, but there was no sign of abnormal tissue that might indicate the complication known as Barrett's esophagus.

Biopsies performed during the EGD confirmed that James did not have Barrett's esophagus. The gastroenterologist recommended that James continue taking his proton-pump inhibitor once a day.

As long as he was taking his medication, James did not have any GERD symptoms. But whenever he stopped taking his medicine, he would quickly have a recurrence of symptoms, usually within a few days.

When lifestyle modifications and over-the-counter antacids or H_2-blockers don't relieve the mild, intermittent symptoms typical of GERD, then prescription medications or surgery may be needed to control GERD symptoms and prevent complications. In this chapter we describe the various options for prescription medications and look at what's involved in surgery for treating GERD.

Prescription Medications for Treating GERD

In a random survey of about 1,000 adults in the United States, only 15 percent of people who regularly used nonprescription H_2-blockers reported complete relief of symptoms. This is probably because the nonprescription H_2-blockers are provided in doses that are only half the starting doses of prescription H_2-blockers, and thus are less likely to provide complete relief. With more than 60 million prescriptions for H_2-blockers and other anti-acid drugs being written by doctors each year, it's clear that a large number of people need prescription medications to control their symptoms.

We recommend that you seek prompt medical attention if you have any of the following symptoms:

* difficult or painful swallowing
* frequent nausea and vomiting
* vomiting of blood
* signs of bleeding from the gastrointestinal tract (either fresh blood or "old" blood in the stools)
* loss of appetite
* weight loss
* feeling full early during meals

Also, if you have any of the unusual symptoms of GERD described in Chapter 3, such as chronic cough or hoarseness, unexplained chest pain, and asthma attacks, you should seek medical advice promptly. And if chronic GERD symptoms suddenly clear up on their own, you will want to make sure the improvement is not due to a complication such as a stricture (see Chapter 8).

Even if you do not have any of these "alarm" symptoms or any unusual symptoms at all, if you are not getting relief from OTC medications or if you have to take more than the recommended doses of such medications to relieve your symptoms, then you may need to visit your doctor for an evaluation and treatment. Most people prefer not to devote time or money to a simple problem that will sometimes clear up by itself, so the question is, How will you know when it's appropriate to seek medical attention? If, for example, you find that you need to take more than the recommended dose of OTC medication only temporarily, such as for a few days or a week, and then your symptoms resolve, this means that your disease is probably not getting worse, and it is probably safe not to see your doctor. We would say, however, that *persistent symptoms or decreased response to formerly effective treatment beyond a week or two* warrants investigation by a medical professional.

The types of testing that are routinely performed to evaluate GERD are described in Chapter 4. But keep in mind that many (if not most) physicians, after reassuring themselves that a patient's symptoms are typical of GERD and do not fall into the "alarming" category, will simply prescribe anti-acid medications as a therapeutic trial, and not order any diagnostic tests unless the patient does not respond to a prescription medication or unless the patient's symptoms return after initially successful treatment. This approach to treatment is appropriate for the many people whose symptoms will respond to prescription medications, because it spares them unnecessary testing, with its associated inconvenience, discomfort, costs, and risks.

Physicians and other prescribing health professionals (such as nurse practitioners) have a useful armamentarium of drugs when it comes to treating GERD. The three classes of prescription drugs for treating GERD are H_2-blockers, proton-pump inhibitors, and prokinetic agents. All the medicines in a particular class act in similar or identical ways.

The differences among the various members of a single drug class often have to do with potency, duration of effect, and frequency of certain side effects rather than with how they work or what they are used to treat. Often the differences are minor and the drugs are essentially interchangeable when used in equivalent doses.

Because many of the various GERD medications have the same action and effectiveness, the physician often takes cost into consideration when prescribing a medication. Medicines that have been available longer than the life of a U.S. patent (17 years) can be purchased in a *generic* form (that is, not under a brand or trade name), generally at a lower price than a brand-name drug. When a generic form is available, the physician can specify on the prescription that the pharmacy should provide the generic form of the medication rather than the brand name. Generic forms of cimetidine are available now, with ranitidine and omeprazole scheduled to go "off patent" over the next several years. It is not unusual, however, for the physician to prescribe the brand of drug he or she is most familiar with.

H_2-Blockers

The class of drugs known as H_2-blockers includes a variety of these "interchangeable" drugs, several of which are available in both over-the-counter and prescription forms. For people with GERD symptoms that are frequent or severe, or that do not respond to OTC medications, one of the prescription H_2-blockers is usually prescribed for an initial period of four to eight weeks.

The four H_2-blockers approved by the U.S. Food and Drug Administration and their standard doses are:

* cimetidine (Tagamet), 400 mg twice a day
* famotidine (Pepcid), 20 mg twice a day
* nizatidine (Axid), 150 mg twice a day
* ranitidine (Zantac), 150 mg twice a day

In the listed doses, these four H_2-blockers are roughly equivalent in potency, effectiveness, and safety. They are all well tolerated and are among the most frequently prescribed medications in the United States. Different treatment studies show wide variations in the rate of symptom relief and healing of esophagitis (because different studies have different patients with different degrees of severity of disease), but a "ballpark" figure is that half of the patients who receive prescription-strength H_2-blockers experience relief from their GERD symptoms and healing of esophagitis, if present.

Neither OTC nor prescription-strength H_2-blockers are very effective at blocking meal-stimulated acid secretion, however, and this is a common cause of reflux symptoms. Also, people develop a tolerance over time to the acid-blocking effect of OTC and prescription-strength H_2-blockers. This means that a person who initially experiences good relief of GERD symptoms may find only one month later that the relief is not as satisfactory, even if there is no change in the underlying pathophysiology. That is, the disease is not necessarily getting worse, but the medication has become less effective (remember Joe, in Chapter 1). Some people also develop a temporary rebound effect after discontinuing acid-suppressing medications, and *more* acid is produced than formerly; this, of course, can temporarily make GERD symptoms worse. If there is no relief from symptoms, or if there is only incomplete relief, the physician may choose to double the dose of the H_2-blocker or switch to the most potent class of medication used in the treatment of GERD, the proton-pump inhibitors (described below).

Side effects of treatment with H_2-blockers are rare. Cimetidine alone among the four has some potential for interacting with other medications, such as the blood thinner warfarin (Coumadin), the antifungal agent ketoconazole, the antiseizure medicine phenytoin, and the asthma medicine theophylline. For a person taking any of these medicines, one of the other H_2-blockers listed above would generally be recommended instead of cimetidine. If for some reason such a person were taking cimetidine, he or she would need to have frequent blood tests to monitor any changes in the effect of the other medications.

If you are taking an H_2-blocker for GERD and your symptoms are relieved, either at the standard dose (listed above) or at a double dose, the next decision is whether to continue the treatment or to stop. Since it is best not to take medicines unless they are needed, after the initial four to eight weeks of treatment the health care provider will generally recommend stopping the medications. Since many people have only intermittent symptoms of GERD and may never have a problem again (especially if they adhere to the lifestyle modifications described in Chapter 5), it is very reasonable to try a period off medications.

If symptoms recur soon after the medication is discontinued, the doctor may recommend performing an upper endoscopy to assess whether the patient has esophagitis or other complications of GERD, or some other problem such as ulcers. Or the doctor may recommend resuming the previously effective dose of medication every day for an additional four to eight weeks. Either of these courses is reasonable, and the final decision often depends on the age of the patient, the duration of the problem, and the severity of the symptoms when they recur. If the decision is made to resume medication, and if the symptoms again respond to medication, then the doctor may again try to stop or reduce the dose of the medication. If this time the symptoms do not recur, or recur only much later, or recur at very mild levels, then intermittent *symptomatic treatment* is generally the recommended course. (Symptomatic treatment is treatment administered only when there are symptoms, as opposed to long-term treatment, which is ongoing.)

Proton-Pump Inhibitors

For some people, H_2-blockers, even at high doses, are inadequate to control symptoms. In particular, if an upper endoscopy is performed and shows that the person has esophagitis, then the most powerful anti-acid medications, the proton-pump inhibitors, are usually prescribed. The proton-pump inhibitors have been shown to provide better acid suppression, and better and faster-onset symptom control, in severe, H_2-blocker-resistant cases of GERD. In addition, they are more effective and faster at healing GERD-related esophagitis than H_2-blockers. Proton-pump inhibitors are only available with a prescription.

The five FDA-approved proton-pump inhibitors and their standard doses are:

* lansoprazole (Prevacid), 30 mg once a day
* omeprazole (Prilosec), 20 mg once a day
* pantoprazole (Protonix), 40 mg once a day
* rabeprazole (Aciphex), 20 mg once a day
* esomeprazole (Nexium), 40 mg once a day

For GERD or GERD with esophagitis, the usual dose is one tablet or capsule taken once daily. As with the H_2-blockers, for people whose GERD is not well controlled on the standard dose, or whose associated esophagitis does not heal well (perhaps 10 to 20 percent of people with esophagitis), the dose of the proton-pump inhibitors can be doubled or even tripled, usually by increasing the number of times each day the standard dose is taken from once a day to two or three times a day.

The proton-pump inhibitors are generally well tolerated. The most common side effects are headache, dizziness, diarrhea, constipation, fatigue, and abdominal discomfort, but none of these individual symptoms occurs in more than 3 percent of people taking proton-pump inhibitors daily. Some concern was raised a number of years ago about long-term use of proton-pump inhibitors because of an increased rate of a rare tumor (called *carcinoid*) in the stomachs of rats given high doses of proton-pump inhibitors. Fortunately, this has not occurred in human beings, so there is no longer any concern about this for people who need to take proton-pump inhibitors for years. Some proton-pump inhibitors can alter the levels of the blood-thinning medication warfarin (Coumadin), so frequent blood tests to monitor the degree of anticoagulation in the blood may be advisable for someone taking both a proton-pump inhibitor and warfarin.

People who feel better on a medicine like omeprazole or lansoprazole often ask how long they can safely stay on it. In the case of omeprazole, a recent study followed patients treated with omeprazole for 12 continuous years and found no significant adverse effects when the patients were compared with a similar group of patients not treated with omeprazole. Omeprazole has now been available for more than 15 years. Although there were some concerns about the long-term safety of this medication when it was first released, these concerns have been laid to rest with the extensive clinical safety track record that has been amassed around the world.

Lansoprazole has been available in the United States for nearly 10 years, and its safety record is also excellent, although there are no published studies that have looked at the long-term use of lansoprazole, like the study described above for omeprazole. Because omeprazole and lansoprazole are chemically very similar, however, we would expect them to be equally safe.

Pantoprazole is the first proton-pump inhibitor that can be administered intravenously, and it is particularly useful in hospitalized people who cannot take medications by mouth.

Prokinetic Agents

A third class of medicine, used less frequently than H_2-blockers or proton-pump inhibitors, is represented by the prokinetic agent metoclopramide (Reglan). Cisapride (Propulsid), another prokinetic agent, was recently withdrawn from the U.S. market because of an unacceptably high rate of heart rhythm abnormalities associated with its use in susceptible individuals. It is still available from the manufacturer on a very limited basis (on a so-called compassionate-clearance basis) through special programs for patients who have not responded well to any treatment other than cisapride. If you are taking cisapride because you are enrolled in such a special program or because you live outside of the United States, you should not take the following medications at the same time: the antibiotics erythromycin and clarithromycin, the antifungal ketoconazole, the antidepressant nefazodone (Serzone), and the anti-HIV drug Retrovir.

Prokinetic drugs work not by decreasing acid secretion but by improving the clearance of refluxed acid. They are used, alone or in combination with H_2-blockers or proton-pump inhibitors, primarily when heartburn is accompanied by prominent abdominal bloating or fullness, symptoms that may be a sign of impairment in the motility (muscle contractions) of the esophagus or stomach. People with impaired motility often respond to prokinetic agents. Now that cisapride is no longer widely available, the older prokinetic, metoclopramide, is being used instead.

The most common side effects of the prokinetics are loose stools and abdominal cramping, a consequence of the drug's action in increasing the motility of other portions of the GI tract besides the stomach and esophagus. Metoclopramide may also cause neurologic effects, such as disorientation and uncontrolled movement, particularly in older adults and people with diabetes.

New prokinetic agents are being developed, and testing is under way (see Chapter 10). The new agents, we hope, will prove as helpful as the older ones in the treatment of GERD, without the side effects that make the older agents a problem for many people.

Maintenance Therapy

Even when GERD symptoms have been controlled by effective treatment, at least half of all patients will have a recurrence of symptoms within a year after they stop taking H_2-blockers or proton-pump inhibitors. This is because medication that reduces acid secretion or increases acid clearance from the esophagus does not correct the underlying abnormality of a weak lower esophageal sphincter or a disorder of esophageal motility. This situation is similar to the treatment of high blood pressure: stop the medicine, and the blood pressure goes back up. The only way to make sure that symptoms are kept "at bay" is to continue medications indefinitely.

One might assume that the dose of antacid medication needed to eliminate reflux symptoms and heal esophagitis would be higher than the dose needed to prevent a recurrence, since even a partial reduction in acid should make it easier for the natural defenses of the esophagus to prevail against bouts of reflux. Thus, it seems logical that a person could go on a low dose of medication indefinitely, as maintenance therapy in GERD treatment. Unfortunately, for the H_2-blockers "a little acid suppression" appears to be ineffective in eliminating recurrences. Low doses of the proton-pump inhibitors (omeprazole 10 mg or lansoprazole 15 mg once daily, for example) are more effective, but not much more, with only 62 percent of patients in one study staying in remission for a year on low-dose omeprazole therapy. On the other hand, in this same study the standard dose of omeprazole, 20 mg once daily, resulted in 72 percent of patients having no recurrence for a year. In other studies, the standard dose eliminated symptoms in 80 percent and even 100 percent of patients. The addition of cisapride to maintenance proton-pump inhibitor therapy has been shown to decrease the recurrence of both GERD symptoms and erosive esophagitis, but, as noted above, cisapride is no longer a therapeutic option for most patients in the United States.

Most physicians will recommend that patients go on standard-dose maintenance therapy if GERD symptoms recur after stopping treatment with an H_2-blocker or proton-pump inhibitor. Before a patient begins maintenance therapy, normally an upper endoscopy is done (if it has not already been done) to confirm the diagnosis and look for GERD complications such as severe esophagitis and strictures.

Surgery

Alma, 37 years old, first developed heartburn symptoms at age 15. During her late teens and early twenties she routinely took baking soda each night to relieve her symptoms. She usually had to take six or eight Tums or Rolaids tablets each day, as well, to control the burning in her chest. In her early twenties she started taking cimetidine, but after a few years this didn't seem to help anymore, and her family doctor switched her to ranitidine. For the next 10 years she routinely took two to four ranitidine tablets each day. On most days her symptoms of burning and regurgitation were fairly well controlled, but her friends joked that whenever they went out to eat, it was guaranteed that Alma would bring a bottle of Mylanta. She had switched several years before because Mylanta seemed to work faster than Tums. Some weeks she would go through an entire large bottle of the liquid antacid. Her doctor had discussed lifestyle modifications with her, and she did her best to adhere to that advice. Her doctor had also ordered a barium swallow, the results of which were normal.

At age 35, Alma stopped taking ranitidine and started taking omeprazole once a day. At first she felt great—all of her symptoms went away. But after about six months the symptoms returned, and she had to start drinking liquid antacids again. At that point Alma's doctor increased her omeprazole dose to twice a day, and again she was symptom-free. Six months later, however, she was again having severe heartburn nearly every day.

Alma's symptoms remained this way for about a year, and then her doctor advised her to see a specialist in gastroesophageal reflux disease. When Dr. Colin Robinson saw Alma, he was reassured by the fact that she did not have any warning signs of complications. Specifically, she wasn't anemic, wasn't losing weight unintentionally, and didn't have difficulty swallowing. Dr. Robinson asked her to continue the omeprazole twice a day but also asked that she take metoclopramide before each meal and at bedtime. He hoped that this prokinetic agent would help the esophagus empty itself of the acid that was causing inflammation there. The doctor asked her to return in four weeks for a follow-up exam and for an upper endoscopy.

Four weeks later Alma returned—symptom-free. This was the best she had felt since age 15. Her endoscopy showed some esophagitis, but no evidence of Barrett's esophagus. Alma told Dr. Robinson that although she felt great, she was concerned about the price of her medications. They were expensive, and although her insurance company paid for most of them, they were still a burden on her limited income. In addition, she found it difficult to remember to take all of them at the scheduled times, and she was worried about the long-term use of such medications. She also wondered whether she would need to take these medicines for the rest of her life.

Dr. Robinson explained that GERD is a chronic disease, and that it was highly unlikely that her symptoms would go away on their own. He also explained that despite being on high doses of the two best medicines currently available to treat heartburn, she still had evidence on endoscopy of continuing damage. He recommended that Alma see a surgeon to discuss an operation to tighten her lower esophageal sphincter. This surgery would almost certainly mean that she could take much less medicine—even possibly none—and it would address her esophagitis before it became more serious. Her doctor thought surgery would improve Alma's overall quality of life.

When Alma saw the surgeon two weeks later, he spent a lot of time discussing both the risks and the benefits of the surgery. He pointed out that without surgery she would probably need medicines for the rest of her life, and that because she was still having both symptoms and ongoing injury to her esophagus, without surgery she could develop a complication of GERD, such as a stricture or Barrett's esophagus. He recommended that she have both a 24-hour pH probe and an esophageal motility study prior to surgery.

The motility study revealed that Alma's LES had very poor tone. This poor tone meant that the natural barrier between the stomach and the lower esophagus was wide open, and gastric acid could easily pour into the esophagus and cause injury. The motility study also showed that Alma had good muscle strength in the rest of the esophagus and that, if she did have the operation, the esophagus would be strong enough to overcome the new, tighter LES.

The 24-hour pH probe was performed three days after Alma stopped taking metoclopramide. She continued the omeprazole, however, because Dr. Robinson wanted to see if she was still having acid reflux while on a proton-pump inhibitor. This test showed that she had multiple episodes of acid reflux and that she spent nearly 30 percent of her day with acid bathing her esophagus (normal is less than 4 to 5 percent of the day).

Although Alma was a little unsure about the operation at first, those tests confirmed her suspicion that without the surgery, she would need to be on medication for life. Two weeks later she had antireflux surgery, a *laparoscopic Nissen fundoplication* (described later). The procedure went smoothly, and she was discharged from the hospital after an overnight stay.

Alma had a little trouble swallowing the first week after the operation and mostly ate thin soups, yogurt, gelatin, and other soft foods. By two weeks after the operation, however, she felt great. She could eat anything she wanted and stopped all of her medicines. Six months later another EGD was performed to make sure that she didn't have any esophagitis and that Barrett's had not appeared. The test was perfectly normal, and Alma continued to feel great. And she is very pleased that she doesn't have to take medicines anymore.

Medications can effectively treat the vast majority of patients who suffer from GERD. However, because GERD is a chronic disease, many patients need to take medications on a daily basis for years at a time. This is expensive for both the patient and the health care system as a whole: in 1998, over 80 million prescriptions were written to treat conditions associated with stomach acid, at a cost of more than $6 billion. It is estimated that proton-pump inhibitor sales in the year 2001 will be *greater than $12 billion in the United States alone.* In addition to being expensive, medications have the drawback of treating the symptoms of acid reflux disease without addressing the underlying physiological problem of a weak lower esophageal sphincter. Physicians have long sought other treatments, including surgery.

Surgery is an alternative to continually using anti-acid medications. Studies show that surgery provides better symptom relief and healing of esophagitis than standard-dose H_2-blockers. (Data are not yet available comparing surgery with proton-pump inhibitors.) Further, symptom relief after surgery appears to be long-lasting, even permanent.

Surgery for acid reflux disease was first performed in 1951. These early operations required making a large incision in the chest and abdomen. Patients remained in the hospital for a long time to recover from this difficult, "open," surgery. In addition, the complication rate from the surgery was fairly high. Over the years the operation was dramatically refined, and in the last decade an operation called a *Nissen fundoplication,* in which the fundus (the upper part of the stomach, located near the esophagus) is wrapped around the lower esophagus, was developed. (*Fundoplication* means a folding *[plication]* of the fundus.) This surgery strengthens the barrier function of the lower esophagus, preventing gastroesophageal reflux and thus repairing the major abnormality that occurs in people suffering from GERD. And the surgery is now usually performed *laparoscopically* (explained below). Figure 7.1 shows how the esophagus and the stomach appear before and after a Nissen fundoplication.

When compared with previous types of operations performed for GERD, the laparoscopic Nissen fundoplication is much safer, has fewer complications, leads to better acid control, and now usually requires only a one- or two-day hospital stay. Some institutions now perform the surgery as a same-day operation, without any overnight hospital stay. This, too, appears to be safe, although most hospitals require at least an overnight stay to monitor the patient for any early complications from the surgery.

As noted above, today a Nissen fundoplication does not usually require open surgery. The technique has become "closed" because it is performed as laparoscopic surgery. With laparoscopic technology, the surgeon sees and operates through instruments inserted through small

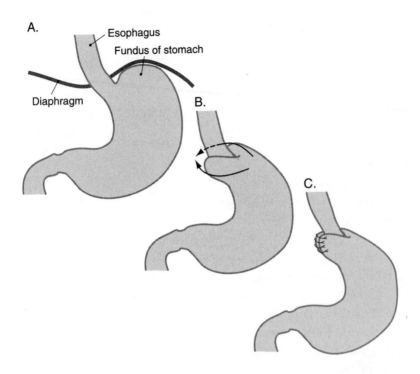

A.

Esophagus

Fundus of stomach

Diaphragm

B.

C.

Figure 7.1. Antireflux surgery. In the most common type of surgery performed, a Nissen fundoplication, the fundus *(A)* is wrapped around the lower esophageal sphincter *(B)* to tighten the sphincter and prevent reflux. It is then sutured *(C)*.

openings in the abdomen rather than through a long incision. Laparoscopic Nissen fundoplication has cut down substantially on the risks, recovery time, and cost of the surgery. General anesthesia is used, and the patient is instructed to stay home from work for one to two weeks after surgery and not to do any heavy lifting.

Nonetheless, laparoscopic surgery is still surgery, and complications do occur in 10 to 15 percent of patients undergoing a laparoscopic Nissen fundoplication. Most complications are minor. The most likely serious complication is *unrecognized perforation* (a hole) in the esophagus, but even this is rare, particularly so when the surgery is performed by a surgeon who has extensive experience in laparoscopic Nissen fundoplication. (When a perforation occurs, a second operation is generally needed.) Other problems after Nissen fundoplication include difficulty burping or belching because the LES is tight, a situation called *gas bloat syndrome*. A more common problem is *dysphagia* (difficulty swallowing) after surgery. Many patients have this problem temporarily in the week or two after surgery, but only about 3 percent of patients have some permanent difficulty swallowing after surgery, and this can sometimes be treated by dilating (stretching) the esophagus.

Laparoscopic Nissen fundoplication initially relieves typical reflux symptoms of heartburn and regurgitation in more than 90 percent of people who have the surgery. As noted below, only patients who have severe or *refractory* (difficult to treat) GERD symptoms or complications of GERD (severe erosive esophagitis, stricture, or Barrett's esophagus) are referred for surgery. Because only people with severe disease have the surgery, this success rate is particularly impressive. The long-term benefits of antireflux surgery may not be quite as striking as the short-term benefits, however. A recent study found that 10 years after undergoing antireflux surgery, nearly 60 percent of patients were taking some form of medication for acid reflux disease. However, 90 percent of those patients stated that they would undergo the operation again, if necessary. Thus, although some form of medication may still be necessary after this surgery, most patients who undergo it are satisfied with the results.

Who, then, should consider having surgery as treatment for GERD? First, only people who have objectively documented, severe GERD or complications of GERD should be considered. Thus, an upper endoscopy and a 24-hour pH study are critical to confirm that GERD is, indeed, the cause of the symptoms. Once a decision is made to pursue surgery, an additional test, esophageal manometry (described in Chapter 4), is also usually performed. It is important to perform this test before surgery to make certain that, other than a weak lower esophageal sphincter, there is sufficient strength (normal motility) in the muscles of the esophagus to propel ingested food through the "wrapped" lower esophagus after the Nissen. If there is some weakness of propulsion, a partial wrap (also called an *incomplete wrap*) may be performed instead of the usual complete, 360-degree, wrap. The LES will not be as tight with this less complete wrap, so the person with decreased motility should still be able to propel food from the esophagus to the stomach. Patients with severe symptoms who do not have severe disease such as erosive esophagitis, stricture, or Barrett's esophagus should be considered for surgery if they are dependent on proton-pump inhibitors to control their symptoms.

Although proton-pump inhibitors appear to be safe for long-term use, the prospect of taking proton-pump inhibitors for life, particularly in people under the age of 50, with the costs ranging from $1,000 to $2,000 per year, may be undesirable. Some people much prefer a one-shot treatment—surgery—over long-term drug treatment, and still others may be referred for surgery because they have difficulty, for any number of reasons, in complying with daily drug treatment. When GERD medications aren't taken faithfully, recurrences and complications increase.

While surgery is an aggressive form of treatment, the results and safety of the procedure are both good. Surgery is a reasonable option for patients with severe, refractory GERD, and for patients with complications of GERD. Of course, anyone who is considering taking this path should have a detailed discussion with his or her primary care physician or gastroenterologist as well as with the surgeon.

In April 2000 the Food and Drug Administration approved two new procedures for use in the United States, both of them variations of the Nissen fundoplication. These procedures are designed to offer permanent solutions to acid reflux disease and are touted as being less invasive than surgery. One is called *endoscopic suturing*, and the other is the *Stretta procedure*. Both of these new procedures are described in Chapter 10. Your gastroenterologist or surgeon will help you decide which is the best procedure for you.

Thus far in this book we have focused almost exclusively on efforts to prevent complications of GERD by recognizing symptoms, diagnosing disease, and treating disease. These issues deserve all the attention we have paid to them; as the saying goes, the best offense is a good defense. So if we can recognize and treat GERD early, we can prevent complications. As we have seen, however, this is not always possible. And for patients who develop complications of GERD, recognizing and treating these complications is a primary concern. In the next part of the book we come to terms with GERD complications: what's involved and what we can do about it.

Part IV

COMPLICATIONS

& SPECIAL SITUATIONS

Chapter 8

Complications of GERD

GERD can be physically distressing, emotionally wearing, and in some patients both physically and emotionally debilitating, but for most people it is merely annoying and does not pose a serious health risk. The majority of people who suffer from only occasional episodes of heartburn can treat their symptoms effectively with over-the-counter antacids or one of the non-prescription-strength H_2-blockers. These people rarely develop complications from GERD. On the other hand, about 10 percent of people with symptomatic GERD—approximately 6 million of the more than 60 million Americans who have heartburn symptoms each month—develop a complication from this disease.

As we noted in Chapter 2, each day, in every person, a small amount of stomach acid refluxes into the esophagus. Most people are completely unaware of this normal process, called *physiologic reflux*. Physiologic reflux does not injure the lining of the esophagus, because when this normal reflux occurs, just a small amount of acid sits in the esophagus for only a brief time. But as we have seen, persistent reflux of caustic gastric secretions into the esophagus over a long period of time, or even brief episodes of reflux with large amounts of acid, *can* injure the lining of the esophagus.

When heartburn persists despite consistent use of over-the-counter or even prescription-strength medications, one or more of the esophageal complications of GERD may develop. The same is true when someone chooses to ignore the problem of recurrent heartburn (perhaps dismissing it as "just one of those things"), or when someone has asymptomatic GERD. One of the biggest challenges for physicians who treat people with GERD, then, is to identify those who are at risk for developing a GERD complication such as esophagitis, esophageal stricture, bleeding, Barrett's esophagus, or esophageal cancer (which sometimes develops when Barrett's esophagus is not diagnosed early enough or treated appropriately).

Unfortunately, identifying people who are likely to develop complications is not as straightforward as it sounds. Logically, one might assume that the person with the most severe symptoms would be at greatest risk of developing a complication. But as we discussed in Chapter 3, symptoms are not a useful predictor of the severity of this disease. Moreover, as many as one-third of patients who have difficulties related to GERD, or who develop complications, have never experienced classic heartburn symptoms. From these patients, we know that it's possible to feel fine even with severe GERD. This means that although most people who develop complications of GERD have severe and intractable classic GERD symptoms, it is entirely possible for someone to develop complications without symptoms (see Chapters 3 and 4).

The chance of any one person developing a complication from acid reflux disease is estimated to be less than 10 percent during his or her lifetime. The risk of complications increases the longer the symptoms persist, particularly when the symptoms are not adequately treated or are not controlled, even by adequate treatment. Thus, the type of person who is most likely to develop a complication is older, with longstanding and relatively severe GERD.

A person who ignores severe symptoms of acid reflux, or who has symptoms that persist despite regular use of medications, is more likely to develop a complication than a person whose symptoms are well controlled by medications. If you have severe GERD symptoms that are resistant to medications, or if you have difficulty swallowing, pain with swallowing, bleeding, or chronic coughing or wheezing, then you need to see your doctor immediately. Even if you have GERD symptoms that are well controlled with over-the-counter medications, we recommend that you discuss these symptoms with your doctor at your next office visit.

People with GERD can increase their chances of identifying complications early by keeping a careful watch on the pattern of their symptoms. A change in the usual pattern of GERD symptoms may be the sign of a complication. While it is logical to assume that if typical symptoms get worse, then a complication may develop, the ironic fact is that *spontaneous improvement in symptoms* (that is, improvement not related to taking a new medication or to taking an old medication more consistently) *may also be a sign of trouble.* This is what happened to Andrew.

Andrew, 55 years of age, had been having a problem with frequent heartburn for many years. His heartburn had been diagnosed 15 years earlier by his primary care physician as likely being due to GERD, and Andrew began taking Zantac, a prescription-strength H_2-blocker, at that time. The Zantac worked well, and he took it every day, consistently, for several years.

Then Andrew decided to test whether he really needed the medication, and he began to take it only when he had symptoms. When the prescription refills ran out, rather than see his doctor, Andrew switched to the nonprescription, over-the-counter, strength of his medication. That was two years ago. While the over-the-counter version didn't work as well as the prescription medicine, Andrew had heartburn "only" two or three times a week, on average, and the OTC pills usually cleared the symptoms up within a few hours.

Over the past several months, Andrew began to notice that his attacks of heartburn were occurring less frequently and were less severe. He was taking almost no over-the-counter medicine, and he thought this was a sign that his GERD had disappeared. But then Andrew developed chest discomfort, with a feeling that solid food was getting stuck behind his breastbone. If he drank some water, the food would eventually pass and the discomfort would disappear.

Andrew was worried enough by his trouble swallowing that he visited his family physician, who recommended that Andrew see a gastroenterologist. A week later, the gastroenterologist performed an upper endoscopy. The EGD showed that Andrew had a stricture in the lower esophagus. Andrew's chronic acid irritation had produced this condition. After the stricture was treated by dilating (stretching) the esophagus, Andrew noticed a dramatic improvement in his swallowing, but his heartburn seemed to get worse until he again began taking his prescription medication regularly.

Paying careful attention to the severity, frequency, and type of symptoms can give you and your physician early warning of the development of a complication of simple GERD. Clearly, the best course of action is to avoid GERD, whenever possible, by making correct decisions about what and when to eat. Next best is to treat GERD so that complications do not develop. And, finally, if complications do develop, treatment needs to be aggressive, maybe even including surgery. The good news is that GERD can often be avoided and that even if a person develops GERD, it is often possible to avoid complications. And if complications do develop, they are rarely life-threatening. The mortality (death rate) in people who have GERD and who develop a complication of acid reflux disease is estimated to be less than 1 patient in 1 million.

In this chapter we will look more closely at the esophageal complications of GERD and review their symptoms—as well as what can be done to avoid them and what can be done to treat them. Complications of GERD in the esophagus can be divided into two general categories, based on how quickly they develop in response to episodes of acid reflux. Some complications are *acute,* meaning that they develop rapidly over hours, days, or weeks. Other complications are *chronic,* meaning that they take longer to develop, usually months or years. Chronic complications occur as a result of extended or repeated episodes of acid reflux.

Esophagitis

When the esophagus is injured, the lining of the esophagus becomes irritated and inflamed (reddened). This condition, called *esophagitis,* affects between 2 and 4 percent of the U.S. adult population and up to 5 percent of people over age 55. It is the most common form of esophageal injury, and it is usually mild. The symptoms of esophagitis are generally indistinguishable from the symptoms of GERD without esophagitis: primarily heartburn and regurgitation. Mild esophagitis generally heals on its own, but the process of healing can be speeded up by treating symptoms with H_2-blockers or antacids. These agents neutralize acid that could reinjure the esophagus while it is healing and is most vulnerable to further injury. Mild esophagitis appears on endoscopy as a redder, irritated part of the esophagus; in some cases the redness and irritation cover the entire esophagus.

A more severe form of esophagitis sometimes develops when on-going GERD brings the mucosal lining of the esophagus into repeated contact with refluxed acid. A person with this form of esophagitis may develop an erosion or ulcer in the esophagus. An *erosion* is a superficial sore on the lining of the esophagus, while an *ulcer* is an erosion that has penetrated deeper into the lining of the esophagus. Between 2 and 7 percent of people with GERD develop an esophageal ulcer or erosion.

If stomach acid is suppressed during the healing phase, esophageal ulcers usually heal without any long-term complications. Rarely (in less than 2 percent of people with GERD), however, esophagitis is so acute that severe bleeding occurs, or an ulcer or erosion rup-tures through the entire thickness of the esophagus. A hole that goes through the entire wall of the esophagus is called a *perforation*. This is a medical emergency and may require surgery. It is a potentially fatal complication of acid reflux but fortunately is very, very rare.

About half of all people with GERD who have an upper endoscopy will be found to have evidence of esophagitis. This very large pro-portion is probably an overestimate of the true proportion of people with GERD who have esophagitis, because only the sickest patients undergo endoscopy in the first place. This overestimate is due to a factor called *ascertainment bias*. This bias arises because we are not ex-amining a random sampling of all patients with GERD but, instead, are examining a population of patients with unusual symptoms or symp-toms that are difficult to control. Therefore, the proportion of people with GERD who actually have esophagitis is probably much lower than half of all people with GERD.

The natural history, or natural progression, of esophagitis, is be-lieved to be approximately as follows:

* About 45 percent of people with esophagitis have it as an isolated episode: the person has it once and is then cured.
* Another 30 percent have recurrences of their esophagitis, but the recurrences are nonprogressive: the subsequent episodes do not increase in severity.
* The remaining 25 percent of people treated for esophagitis may have recurrent, progressive disease: the subsequent episodes may be more severe, or they may be associated with other complications of GERD such as strictures, bleeding, or Barrett's esophagus (all discussed below).

Doctors currently have little way of knowing which patients are most likely to suffer from recurrent or progressive episodes of esophagitis. Also, at the present time the diagnosis of esophagitis can be made only through imaging studies like endoscopy or upper GI x-ray series, and can be made with *certainty* only by examining a biopsy of the affected portion of the esophagus under a microscope. Doctors do know that esophagitis, like all complications of GERD, is more likely to occur, and to recur or progress, in people who have untreated GERD or poorly controlled GERD symptoms and, as noted above, in people over the age of 55.

Esophagitis can also develop in people who do not have GERD. A fungus called *Candida albicans* can cause esophagitis, for example. Also, when pills, especially potassium, tetracycline, or iron supplements, accidentally stick in the esophagus, they can injure it and cause esophagitis.

Treating Esophagitis

Treating esophagitis, as well as preventing the recurrence and progression of the disease, means effectively controlling acid reflux into the esophagus, whether with medications that reduce or eliminate acid, or with surgery to prevent acid from refluxing into the esophagus. For almost every patient, controlling reflux not only effectively controls the symptoms of GERD but also helps eliminate episodes of esophagitis.

As we noted earlier in this book, over-the-counter antacids and H_2-blockers often are effective and are the first line of treatment for simple GERD. Mild esophagitis also generally clears up with this approach. People with severe esophagitis, however, need to be treated with the more powerful proton-pump inhibitors, because severe esophagitis does not respond as well or as rapidly to treatment as uncomplicated GERD does.

An initial 12-week course of treatment with a proton-pump inhibitor—omeprazole, lansoprazole, rabeprazole, esomeprazole, or pantoprazole—is the standard treatment for severe esophagitis. A second endoscopy is often performed, after the initial course of therapy, to confirm that the esophagitis has healed. Then, a decision is made about what type and dose of medication is most likely to prevent recurrence of esophagitis. A lower dose of the proton-pump inhibitor or a switch to a less powerful medication like one of the H_2-blockers is generally the recommended maintenance treatment after the initial bout of esophagitis is healed. Because almost half of those who suffer an attack of GERD with esophagitis have no recurrences or progression of the esophagitis, it may be advisable to use a less powerful maintenance medication after a first attack. If the esophagitis *does* return for a second attack while the person is taking the less powerful medication (or if the prescribed maintenance treatment was not being taken regularly), then maintenance treatment with a proton-pump inhibitor is needed from that point on. Such maintenance therapy should be continued indefinitely, not only to help prevent recurrences but also to help prevent other complications.

Strictures

Remember James, from the previous chapter? Two years after his first upper endoscopy, James began to have trouble swallowing solid food.

James's difficulty with swallowing food began slowly, and at first he hardly noticed it. In fact, only when he was eating steak did he have the sensation of food sticking behind his breastbone. Drinking water or other liquids would immediately relieve the sensation of the food sticking. Without really ever thinking about it, James altered his diet, eliminating steak, chicken, and other hard-to-swallow foods in favor of "softer" foods. With time, however, the sensation grew more frequent and began to occur even with softer foods, like rice, pasta, and bananas.

Remarkably enough, James was not having any problems with his previous symptoms of heartburn and regurgitation, so he was not inclined to take his GERD medication. In addition, he did not seek out the advice of his primary care physician or gastroenterologist when he initially noted difficulty swallowing solid food. James admitted that he was "just tired" of seeing doctors.

When he began to notice that even softer foods seemed to get held up behind his breastbone, however, James consulted his gastroenterologist again. The gastroenterologist was concerned about these new symptoms and decided to perform an EGD, as he had done two years earlier. This time the endoscopy showed that James had developed a stricture just above the level of the lower esophageal sphincter.

Fortunately, the biopsy of the stricture showed there was no malignancy. It was a peptic stricture (one caused by acid reflux) and responded to dilation. The somewhat unpleasant experience of a biopsy followed by dilation gave James all the motivation he needed to remember to take his medication. And once he began taking his medication regularly again, he had no further GERD symptoms and no trouble with swallowing.

There are two lessons here that bear repeating. The first is that complications of GERD commonly occur despite the relative or total absence of continuing symptoms of GERD. The second is that these complications can usually be prevented by taking medications as prescribed.

Some medical studies report that nearly 10 percent of patients who visit their doctors because of heartburn symptoms already have a stricture. Esophagitis is the leading cause of peptic stricture in the esophagus. Pill-induced injury (most commonly from potassium tablets), inherited strictures and rings, and cancer of the esophagus are less common causes.

Let's detour briefly to say something about esophageal rings, technically called *Schatzki's B rings*. A Schatzki's B ring is a very thin rim of tissue—like a simple wedding ring—that develops in the lower esophagus above the gastroesophageal junction. It's not entirely clear why such rings develop, but many physicians believe they develop in response to acid reflux. A person who has an esophageal ring may occasionally get solid food temporarily stuck in the esophagus. This may happen at a social event or at a restaurant with friends, when the person is busy talking and drinking and may not be paying attention to cutting up and chewing his or her food carefully. During one of these episodes, a large piece of meat may become lodged above a ring in the lower esophagus. Sometimes this food passes through the ring by itself, but sometimes people must try to force it down by drinking water. If it still won't pass, the food must be vomited back up. This situation is different from a choking episode, when someone has to use the Heimlich maneuver to eject food from the windpipe because the person can't breathe. A ring is usually easily treated by dilating the esophagus (see below) and breaking the ring open. The ring may develop again, however; about half of treated patients will need a second dilation.

As noted in Chapter 3, peptic strictures develop in the lower esophagus because of repeated injury from acid. Repeated injury and recurrent inflammation due to acid reflux leads to the formation of scar tissue, which creates a thickened, narrowed area in the lower esophagus (see photo and Figure 8.1). This situation is similar to a skin abrasion that is repeatedly injured and never allowed to heal properly. Eventually it will form a scar. The same thing can happen on the inside of the esophagus. However, when a scar forms here, it may lead to a narrowing of the esophagus. This narrowing is called a *stricture.*

A stricture is made up of bands of fibrous tissue under the lining of the esophagus. One clear sign of a stricture is when a person is having difficulty swallowing solid foods. Only someone with a severe stricture will also have trouble swallowing liquids. And, more seriously, a person may have a *food impaction,* which means a blockage of the esophagus caused by food getting stuck at the stricture so that nothing else can get by—in the worst cases, not even saliva. At the other extreme, about one-fourth of people who are found to have GERD-related strictures do not report having symptoms like heartburn or regurgitation. For them, the stricture appears to come out of the blue.

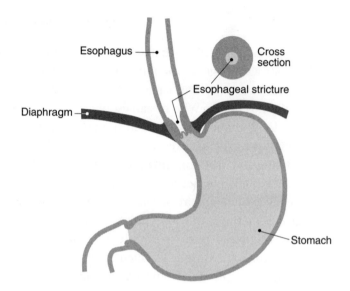

Figure 8.1. Esophageal stricture. If acid refluxes from the stomach into the lower esophagus over many years, inflammation may occur repeatedly. This chronic inflammation eventually develops into scar tissue called a *stricture*. The cross section demonstrates how the stricture decreases the diameter of the esophagus, thus increasing the probability that food will get stuck.

To diagnose a peptic stricture, the physician may order a barium swallow (described in Chapter 4). When seen on an x-ray, most strictures are one-half to two inches in length, are smooth and symmetrical, and are located at the gastroesophageal junction, at the lower end of the esophagus, just above the stomach. During the barium swallow the radiologist may ask the patient to swallow a special barium pill of a predetermined size, to help get an idea of how narrow the stricture is.

The doctor may also refer the patient to a gastroenterologist, if the doctor is concerned about the possibility of a stricture. The patient will probably also be scheduled for an esophagogastroduodenoscopy (EGD, or upper endoscopy) so that the doctor can directly inspect the esophagus, to make sure that the person does not have Barrett's esophagus or cancer in addition to the stricture (40 percent of people with an esophageal stricture also have Barrett's). Biopsies of the stricture can be taken during this procedure, and if necessary the stricture can be dilated at the same time (see below).

Treating Strictures

Treatment of strictures usually requires the use of both medication and esophageal dilation. Medications are prescribed to suppress stomach acid and prevent further esophageal irritation and inflammation. H_2-blockers may be used, but we usually recommend daily or twice-daily proton-pump inhibitors. Several studies have shown that these medications decrease the chance of a stricture developing, and hence lessen the need for esophageal dilation.

Esophageal dilation is a technique that at first glance might seem barbaric. The French term for this procedure is *bougienage* (boo-jee-NAHZH), which certainly makes the procedure sound gentler. To dilate, or stretch, the narrowed area of the esophagus, smooth, rigid rubber or metal dilators called *bougies* (BOO-jees) are inserted into the esophagus. Dilation is usually done during an EGD that is being performed for diagnostic purposes. As noted in Chapter 4, generally the patient has received some type of medication intravenously to help him or her relax. The back of the throat is also usually sprayed with anesthetic to numb it and prevent gagging or choking. The patient is usually asked to sit up or lie back at a 45-degree angle, with the head held slightly forward. The dilator is then carefully lubricated and slid over the tongue, into the back of the throat, and down the esophagus. The gastroenterologist may perform this procedure two or three times in one session, to slowly and safely stretch the esophagus with progressively wider bougies. Instead of using a solid rubber or metal dilator, some doctors dilate the stricture with a balloon that is inflated in the esophagus. Most patients with esophageal strictures need several sessions to dilate the esophagus to the greatest extent possible.

Esophageal dilation is very safe when done gradually. There is a small chance of bleeding from the procedure. The risk of perforation (tearing the esophagus) is estimated at less than 1 percent (1 patient in 100). In some patients the stricture is so narrow and so scarred that dilation cannot be safely performed, or cannot make the esophagus wide enough to restore normal swallowing. For these patients, surgery is usually recommended.

Bleeding

A person with GERD may begin bleeding from the esophagus at any time, and with no warning symptoms, not even heartburn. Bleeding occurs when *erosive esophagitis* (esophagitis that is severe enough to cause an erosion or an ulcer) affects an area that contains blood vessels, or when the esophagitis is severe enough to make the lining of the esophagus very fragile (*friable* is the medical term for this easy bruising of the tissues).

Bleeding may be sudden *(acute)* or gradual and persistent *(chronic)*. In an *acute bleeding episode,* when an artery or vein becomes disrupted by the inflammation of esophagitis, the person may vomit red blood or blood that has been digested by stomach acid (the latter is dark in color and has the appearance of coffee grounds). The blood in an acute bleeding episode may also appear as blood in the stool, either with or without the vomiting of blood. When large volumes of blood travel through the stomach, the acid in the stomach turns the stools black and tarry in appearance. Such stools are often very foul-smelling. (Small volumes of blood do not turn the stools black and can be detected only by a special stool test that involves a chemical reaction and change in color of an indicator paper when the blood reacts with an indicator solution.)

Acute bleeding should be viewed as a medical emergency. Going immediately to an emergency room is the wisest course of action, as there is little that can be done in the doctor's office for most people with acute bleeding from the GI tract. Acute bleeding may require a blood transfusion to replace the lost blood. Acute bleeding, even in someone who is known to have esophagitis, is not always caused by esophagitis, so an upper endoscopy is usually performed to identify the source of the bleeding. (Instead of esophagitis-related bleeding, the EGD may reveal, for example, bleeding from a duodenal ulcer or from abnormal blood vessels in the esophagus. Called *esophageal varices,* these abnormal blood vessels are usually caused by chronic alcohol abuse that has led to cirrhosis of the liver.) Acute bleeding that occurs as a result of esophagitis usually stops spontaneously. When a specific blood vessel is identified on endoscopy as the source of bleeding, it is often possible to stop the bleeding by injecting a substance through the endoscope that causes blood vessels to constrict. Or an electric current can be applied to the bleeding blood vessel to coagulate it.

For most acute bleeding episodes related to GERD-induced esophagitis, no such treatment is needed. Often there is only a small amount of bleeding, or oozing, of some blood from a severely irritated portion of the esophagus. After the source of acute bleeding is diagnosed, a proton-pump inhibitor is generally prescribed to heal the esophagitis.

Chronic bleeding, on the other hand, usually occurs in small amounts at a time, and the blood is not noticed by the patient. Instead, it is usually detected when the stools are tested for invisible *(occult)* blood. Or chronic bleeding from the GI tract may be suspected when there is a drop in the blood count *(anemia),* especially when this anemia is of the kind caused by iron depletion *(iron-deficiency anemia).*

Evaluation of chronic blood loss also usually involves endoscopy. A *colonoscopy* (an examination of the colon by means of an endoscope) may be performed first, to make certain that the iron-deficiency anemia has not been caused by cancer of the colon or some other problem such as a bleeding polyp, an abnormal blood vessel in the colon, or bleeding from diverticular disease. If the colon examination is normal, an upper endoscopy is usually performed to diagnose any esophageal source of bleeding. Chronic bleeding from GERD-related esophagitis is not among the most common causes of blood loss from the GI tract, however, so it is more likely that a non-GERD cause will be identified when an evaluation for chronic anemia or blood-tinged stools is undertaken.

If chronic blood loss related to esophagitis is diagnosed, any resulting anemia is generally treated with iron supplements. A blood transfusion is performed if the anemia is severe. If it is not already being treated, the esophagitis that led to the chronic bleeding will be treated with a proton-pump inhibitor to speed healing. If the esophagitis underlying the blood loss is already being treated with an H_2-blocker, the treatment will be enhanced by switching to a proton-pump inhibitor; if the patient was taking a proton-pump inhibitor at the time the esophageal blood loss was detected, the dose of the proton-pump inhibitor will usually be increased, perhaps from once a day to twice a day.

Barrett's Esophagus

Barrett's esophagus is the complication of GERD that gastroenterologists are most concerned about, because Barrett's is a premalignant (precancerous) condition. Barrett's esophagus is not cancer, but it has a small potential to turn into esophageal cancer. (More information on esophageal cancer appears later in this chapter.) Barrett's esophagus is found in 10 to 15 percent of people with symptomatic GERD, and in over 40 percent of patients with a peptic stricture. Barrett's is more common in older age groups and is usually diagnosed at the age of 55 to 60 years, although most likely the process begins many years earlier but goes unnoticed. This delay in diagnosis is due to the simple fact that Barrett's esophagus, in and of itself, does not cause any symptoms. Three times as many men get Barrett's as women, and it is much more common in Caucasians than in African-Americans.

One study has shown that once Barrett's is present and detected, the area of abnormal tissue does not appear to significantly change its length over time. That is, once it is there, it does not seem to elongate or grow to any significant extent. In addition, once Barrett's is present in the esophagus, it does not usually go away. A gastroenterologist can generally identify this abnormal tissue during endoscopy as a salmon-pink- or red-colored mucosa with fingerlike projections rising up from the junction of the stomach and esophagus and extending upward toward the mouth. It generally stands out against the light-orange color of the normal esophageal mucosa (see photo and Figure 8.2).

When we say that Barrett's esophagus is a premalignant condition and has the potential to develop into esophageal cancer, we must also say that esophageal cancer is uncommon in the United States: fewer than 15,000 people develop esophageal cancer each year in this coun-

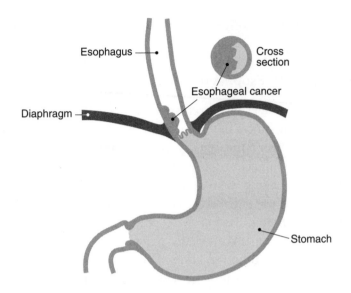

Figure 8.2. Esophageal cancer. An irregularly shaped lesion in the lower esophagus has developed over many years. Such a lesion often does not cause any symptoms until it is large enough to block the movement of food from the esophagus into the stomach. It can be diagnosed with either an EGD or a barium swallow.

try. If you have Barrett's esophagus, your risk of esophageal cancer is 30 to 50 times higher than the risk of a person who does not have Barrett's, but the overall risk is still quite low. It is estimated that a person with Barrett's esophagus has approximately a 0.4 to 1 percent risk of developing esophageal cancer each year he or she has it. This means that a man who is diagnosed with Barrett's esophagus at age 60 might have a lifetime risk of between 10 and 25 percent of developing esophageal cancer, assuming he lives to age 85.

Barrett's esophagus is not passed on genetically from one generation to another. Some types of cancer, such as breast cancer and colon cancer, do tend to develop in families. Someone with a first-degree relative (mother, father, sister, brother) who has colon cancer or breast cancer is at higher risk than the general population to develop that type of cancer. But Barrett's esophagus is not thought to be genetically transmitted. The major risk factor for developing Barrett's esophagus is acid reflux disease.

Treating Barrett's Esophagus

The primary danger of Barrett's esophagus is that it increases the risk of developing cancer of the lower esophagus. The level of this risk likely becomes lower if the underlying GERD and esophagitis are carefully controlled with acid-suppressing medications (especially proton-pump inhibitors) along with lifestyle changes. The current treatment for Barrett's is to use aggressive acid suppression so as to reduce the amount of time that acid is in contact with the esophagus and thus to prevent further injury. We usually recommend the use of daily or twice-daily proton-pump inhibitors. For some patients we may also recommend the use of a prokinetic drug such as metoclopramide to increase motility (muscle contractions) in the esophagus and to help empty any remaining acid.

Cancers detected early are curable, so the most important thing to know here is that the risk of dying from Barrett's-related esophageal cancer can be greatly diminished by maintaining close follow-up medical care and by having regular EGDs performed by a gastroenterologist. For patients with Barrett's esophagus, the gastroenterologist will recommend an upper endoscopy once every six months to once every three years, to make sure cancer is not developing. During the endoscopy, biopsies are taken at several levels of the esophagus. What determines whether a patient has follow-up EGDs every six months, or every three years, or something in between? A variety of factors, including acid reflux symptoms, warning signs of early cancer (such as anemia and unintentional weight loss), and a review of the patient's biopsies from previous endoscopies.

GERD surgery, as described in Chapter 7, is generally not effective in reversing Barrett's esophagus, as studies in patients who have had antireflux surgery generally fail to show reversal in Barrett's esophagus back to the type of mucosa that normally lines the esophagus. Surgery produced an apparent decrease in the length of the region containing Barrett's tissue in only 11 percent of patients. In addition, antireflux surgery will probably not prevent the occurrence of Barrett's.

Experimental treatments are being developed and are in use at

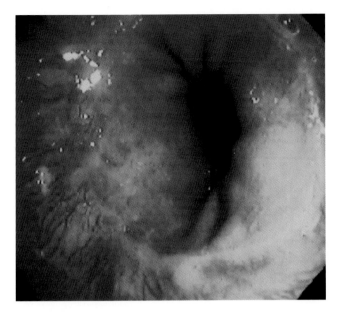

Plate 1. Normal esophagus and normal GE junction. The esophageal mucosa is salmon pink in color, while the gastric mucosa is a deeper pink. The junction of these two different cell types is called the z-line.

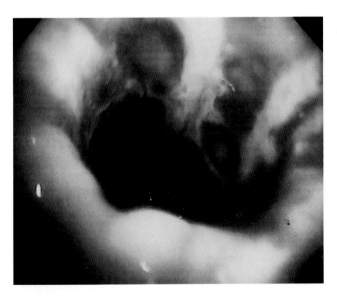

Plate 2. Esophagitis. Severe inflammation with edema and loss of normal vascular pattern in a person with untreated acid reflux.

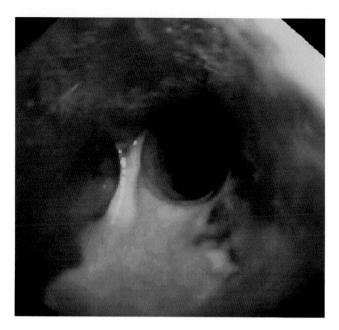

Plate 3. Esophageal stricture. Chronic acid reflux has produced this tight narrowing of the lower esophagus. It is easy to understand how food could get stuck in such a small opening.

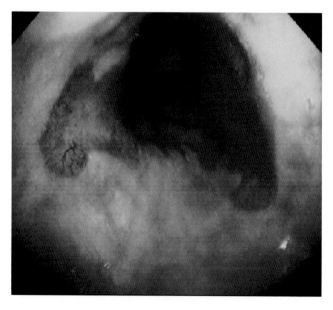

Plate 4. Barrett's esophagus.

some university centers. These treatments seek to destroy the abnormal Barrett's tissue in the esophagus without performing surgery to remove the affected area in the lower esophagus (a major operation). These treatments include laser and laserlike treatments of the tissue, sometimes after it has been made more sensitive to the laser's energy with special chemicals. The patient's primary care physician or gastroenterologist must refer the patient to a center that specializes in this kind of treatment. Furthermore, the results are not yet of proven benefit. (To learn more about the promise of experimental treatments, see Chapter 10.)

Many people with Barrett's (25 percent in one study) have no symptoms of GERD, and some people with GERD symptoms experience improvement or resolution of their symptoms when Barrett's esophagus develops, because the abnormal new columnar-type cells lining the lower esophagus are more resistant to the effects of acid than the normal tissue is. Thus, as is true of strictures, improvement or even absence of symptoms is not necessarily reassuring. Close follow-up with a primary care physician or a gastroenterologist is of the utmost importance in minimizing the complications of GERD. If complications do develop, then it is essential to deal with them early on, when the consequences of the complications are likely to be less severe and more easily treated.

Cancer

Sylvester, a 67-year-old retiree, suffered with GERD symptoms for more than a decade before winding up in the hospital after passing out in a grocery store. He was brought to the emergency room by ambulance. In the ER, Sylvester was found to be dehydrated and anemic, and he complained that he had recently been losing weight and had been feeling weak and light-headed.

Sylvester had smoked cigarettes all his adult life and for many years had drunk alcohol to excess. He had never sought any medical advice or treatment for his symptoms of heartburn and regurgitation. When he did anything about it at all, he took a slug of a liquid antacid and hoped for the best. But in fact, as he told the doctor who took his medical history, his GERD symptoms had recently improved, without treatment.

Sylvester was admitted to the hospital for intravenous fluids and evaluation of his weight loss and anemia. The physical examination revealed that he was *cachectic* (he had a wasted appearance). He also had microscopic amounts of blood in his stools. Because of this, a gastroenterology consultation was requested, and the gastroenterologist recommended that Sylvester undergo an upper endoscopy, in view of the long history of heartburn symptoms, the history of alcohol abuse (a risk factor for the development of esophageal varices), and the anemia.

The endoscopy revealed that Sylvester had a mass growing in the lower part of his esophagus. The mass was biopsied, and cancerous cells were found. The cancer was adenocarcinoma of the lower esophagus. There was also evidence of inflammation and Barrett's esophagus in the area. This combination of findings suggested strongly that Sylvester's cancer had developed in an area of Barrett's esophagus that had formed as a result of acid reflux disease over many years.

The risk of esophageal cancer is thought to be increased in people with chronic GERD and, as we have discussed, is markedly increased in people with the premalignant complication of Barrett's esophagus. A recent study published in the *New England Journal of Medicine* found that the risk of esophageal cancer was almost eight times higher in people who experienced symptoms of heartburn or regurgitation at least once a week than it was in people who did not experience these symptoms. For those with nighttime heartburn symptoms, the risk was 11 times that of people with no symptoms. Finally, people with GERD who had suffered from severe symptoms for at least 20 years were found to have a risk of developing cancer of the esophagus more than 40 times the risk of people without GERD at all. As we mentioned earlier, GERD with Barrett's esophagus dramatically increases the risk of cancer of the lower esophagus; many people with Barrett's have severe symptoms, but a significant percentage have mild symptoms or no symptoms at all.

As noted above, fewer than 15,000 people develop esophageal cancer each year in the United States. Yet the incidence of cancer of the lower esophagus and upper stomach has been increasing since the 1970s in this country, and has risen more sharply than the incidence of any other type of cancer. The rate of esophageal cancer is now six to eight times higher than it was in the 1970s, even after adjusting for the increases in population and the aging of the U.S. population. World-wide, esophageal cancer is the eighth most common form of cancer.

The two major types of esophageal cancer are *adenocarcinoma* and *squamous cell carcinoma*. Squamous cell carcinoma does not seem to be associated with Barrett's esophagus. Instead, people with other risk factors, such as tobacco and alcohol use, seem to get this kind of cancer. Adenocarcinoma, however, *is* associated with Barrett's esophagus. The process in adenocarcinoma appears to be as follows: The normal lining cells of the esophagus are replaced with a new type of cell. More specifically, the normal stratified squamous epithelium of the esophagus is replaced with simple columnar epithelium. This replacement of one cell type by another, a process in this case called *intestinal metaplasia,* occurs in response to repeated episodes of acid reflux injuring the esophagus. Over time, this new type of epithelium may slowly change and transform, and cancer may develop. Fortunately, this process is quite slow, and these changes can usually be identified if biopsies are taken during endoscopy.

Treating Cancer

Unfortunately, cancer of the esophagus that develops in someone with GERD or GERD with Barrett's esophagus, if not detected at an early stage, is usually fatal within a couple of years or, sometimes, months. If the cancer is detected early enough, surgery can be performed and may cure the cancer. Cure is possible only through radical surgery and only if the cancer is found not to have spread widely beyond the lower esophagus. Further information on this complicated topic can best be obtained from an experienced gastroenterologist or surgeon.

Other treatments for esophageal cancer are *palliative treatments,* which means that they are designed not to cure the cancer but to relieve symptoms caused by the cancer, such as the inability to eat solids, or even liquids, when the passageway for nourishment is narrowed because the cancerous tumor is growing inward from the lining of the esophagus or upper stomach. Thus, chemotherapy and radiotherapy are not used to cure esophageal cancer, but they are sometimes of value in reducing the rate of spread and providing palliative treatment.

The most effective palliation is provided by endoscopic techniques that dilate and hold open the area of the esophagus that is becoming closed off by the growth of the tumor. After dilation, wire cages (called *stents*) are sometimes placed in the esophagus through the endoscope to preserve the person's ability to swallow liquids and solids for as long as possible. This, too, is a palliative treatment, not a cure, because it does not stop the spread of the cancer, but it does make it easier for the person to swallow and in that way helps to prevent malnutrition.

Of course, esophageal carcinoma is a dreaded complication of GERD. It must be emphasized that it is an uncommon complication, however, and it can be treated if detected early. People with Barrett's esophagus are at particularly high risk and should periodically undergo a screening endoscopy under the direction of a gastroenterologist.

Our discussion in this book so far has focused on the diagnosis and treatment of GERD in the general population. But GERD affects some groups of people in special ways. In the next chapter we turn to these special populations of GERD patients—children, pregnant women, elderly people, and the bed-bound—and the precautions and treatments that apply specifically to them.

Chapter 9

GERD in Children, Pregnant Women, the Older Patient, and the Bed-Bound

In this book we have noted that people with asthma may find their asthma symptoms getting worse during episodes of GERD, and we have briefly described how the body changes of pregnancy can cause GERD, but for the most part we have looked at how GERD affects otherwise healthy adults. This chapter, however, is dedicated to looking closely at GERD not in the average healthy adult but in special populations: children, pregnant women, older people, and people who are confined to bed. If you belong to one of these groups, there are a number of special requirements and precautions you need to be aware of if you have GERD.

Children

We don't usually think of infants or small children as suffering from acid reflux disease, but GERD is thought to affect a large number of infants and toddlers younger than 2 years of age. Of course, young children can't tell us whether they are having heartburn or regurgitation. Instead, we rely on symptoms or changes in behavior or feeding to help identify the problem. This means we don't know how common the disorder actually is in young children. One study revealed that nearly 20 percent of parents believe that their infant has a problem with regurgitation, although most of these infants never undergo any type of evaluation for the problem. Another study reported that as many as 8 percent of children aged 3 to 17 have acid reflux disease but that few of these children were treated for the disease with medications.

The infant or young child who constantly regurgitates or spits up may very well be suffering from acid reflux disease. Such infants generally bring up two or three teaspoons of formula several times a day. Most infants do not appear to have any other symptoms, and they continue to eat well and gain weight. There is usually no need to treat these infants, because they usually outgrow the spitting up by the time they reach their first birthday. But infants who regurgitate and begin to lose weight usually need medication to treat their acid reflux. They may also require a diagnostic test to fully investigate what's causing their symptoms. (Infants or very young children with weight loss and vigorous vomiting may have GERD, or, less commonly, they may have a condition called *pyloric stenosis*. In this condition, the pylorus—the muscular ring between the stomach and duodenum—is so tight that food cannot empty out of the stomach properly, and it comes back up in what is called *projectile vomiting*. This condition must be corrected with surgery. Other conditions that may masquerade as GERD include malrotation of the gut, gastroparesis, and a connection between the trachea and esophagus called a *fistula*.)

In addition to spitting up and in some cases losing weight, infants with GERD may refuse to eat or take a bottle. They may initially seem to be hungry at feeding time but then become fussy or irritable during feeding, as the food or formula irritates their inflamed esophagus and causes pain. Infants may refuse to take any more formula by pushing the bottle away, clenching their lips, turning their head away, or arching their back. Parents may confuse these episodes of GERD with colic, or they may think their infant is just tired, but when this behavior coincides with the onset of feeding, the diagnosis of GERD needs to be strongly considered.

Other symptoms of acid reflux in children include a chronic cough, new onset or worsening of asthma, choking, hoarseness, difficulty swallowing, or recurrent wheezing or pneumonia. Some children with GERD may be labeled irritable or may be diagnosed with "failure to thrive." Some infants may just have a very nonspecific symptom of GERD, such as arching their back.

Diagnostic tests for acid reflux disease in infants are the same as those used in adults. Barium swallows, upper GI series, upper endoscopy, 24-hour pH probes—all can safely be performed in infants and small children. These procedures are much less likely to be routinely performed in children than adults, however, because most children outgrow their symptoms or respond rapidly to medical therapy. When the diagnosis is in doubt, when warning signs such as difficult or painful swallowing, weight loss, or anemia appear, or when symptoms persist despite medications, diagnostic testing is appropriate.

Treatment for GERD in infants and children usually starts with some simple changes in feeding patterns. First, we recommend adding rice cereal to the formula, to help thicken it. Two to three teaspoons of rice cereal added to each ounce of formula usually makes the formula thick enough to help it stay down. Second, infants should be fed in an upright position, and they should be held upright or propped up in an infant seat for 15 to 20 minutes after feeding, to minimize regurgitation. Finally, neither babies nor toddlers should be bounced or jiggled up and down after feeding, because this may cause them to regurgitate. Elevating the head of the bed to minimize acid reflux has *not* been shown to be helpful in infants. On the subject of sleeping, while the older view was that after feeding, the infant should be placed on his or her stomach for sleeping, the recent information on sudden infant death syndrome (SIDS) has led to the recommendation that a child sleep on his or her back. We do not recommend placing children on their stomach after feeding.

If babies continue to spit up, have difficult feeding times, or remain irritable despite being fed as recommended above, then many doctors recommend a trial of medications. The medications used to treat GERD in adults are also used to treat children, although the doses are closely adjusted for the smaller body weight and different metabolism of infants and children. Over-the-counter antacids should be used in infants and children only after consulting with the child's doctor. Antacids should not be taken continuously by children, nor should they be taken even intermittently for longer than two months without, again, consulting the child's doctor. These guidelines are important because all medications given to a child should be closely monitored by a child's doctor. They are also important because it's essential to avoid both undertreating severe reflux disease in an infant or child and overlooking other diseases with symptoms similar to those of acid reflux disease. An infant or child who is taking antacids (under a doctor's supervision) and whose symptoms are not responding to the medication should be evaluated again, perhaps including a diagnostic test for GERD and other gastrointestinal disorders.

Both H_2-blockers and proton-pump inhibitors can safely be taken by children. Again, over-the-counter H_2-blockers should not be given to children without first consulting the child's doctor. H_2-blockers suppress gastric acid and effectively control symptoms in most children with GERD. Many of the H_2-blockers are available in liquid form by prescription, which makes the medications easier to give to children who can't or won't swallow pills. If symptoms persist, the doctor may want to prescribe a prokinetic medication such as metoclopramide along with the H_2-blocker. An H_2-blocker to suppress gastric acid plus a prokinetic agent to help empty the esophagus and stomach more rapidly and efficiently is a very effective combination. Finally, the child's doctor may decide to use a proton-pump inhibitor such as omeprazole or lansoprazole instead of an H_2-blocker or prokinetic agent. Omeprazole can be specially formulated into a liquid suspension, while lansoprazole can be mixed in with applesauce. This approach is generally effective, and it eliminates the need to give multiple doses of multiple medications. Again, if the infant's or child's symptoms do not respond to medications, further investigation into the cause of the symptoms is called for.

Just like adults, children can have complications of acid reflux disease or have atypical symptoms of GERD, such as severe asthma. Several studies have shown that when children with asthma and reflux disease are treated aggressively for their acid reflux, their asthma often gets better as well. If a child's doctor believes that a child's asthma is severe, and that acid reflux is a critical factor in the symptoms of the asthma, then the best treatment may be to correct the problem surgically. A recent study from a referral center for children with asthma demonstrated that Nissen fundoplication not only treated reflux disease in children with asthma but also dramatically improved their asthma. The surgical treatment has the added benefit of eliminating or reducing the need to take daily medications for acid reflux.

Pregnant Women

Of the many changes of pregnancy, one of the most common is heartburn. Many women complain of developing heartburn symptoms for the first time during pregnancy, or they complain that their heartburn symptoms become worse during pregnancy. Several studies have demonstrated that daily heartburn is more likely to occur in pregnant women than in the general population. One study showed that 25 percent of pregnant women had daily heartburn, compared with 7 to 10 percent of nonpregnant women. In addition, heartburn is more likely to occur as pregnancy progresses from the first to the second to the third trimester. Of 607 pregnant women who completed questionnaires throughout their pregnancies, only 22 percent complained of heartburn in the first trimester of pregnancy, while 39 percent had chronic heartburn in the second trimester, and 72 percent had heartburn during the third trimester.

Is there any way to predict which women will develop heartburn during pregnancy? Yes. Women who have a history of heartburn before becoming pregnant have the greatest likelihood of having heartburn during pregnancy. There is some evidence, too, that symptoms are more likely to occur with multiple births (twins or triplets) than with single births. Heartburn also appears to be more common in subsequent pregnancies if it was present during the first pregnancy. Surprisingly, the amount of weight gained during pregnancy does not appear to have anything to do with whether the woman will develop heartburn.

Pregnant women get heartburn for the same reason anyone else does: the lower esophageal sphincter relaxes too frequently or for an abnormally long period of time. The prolonged or inappropriate relaxation of the LES allows caustic stomach acid to reflux into the esophagus and cause damage. Other factors, such as delayed stomach emptying and decreased esophageal motility (muscle contractions), may also play a role. We know that the muscle tone or pressure of the LES is lower in pregnant women who have reflux symptoms than in pregnant women who do not have symptoms. In addition, the pressure in the LES continues to decrease as the pregnancy progresses. (LES pressures return to prepregnancy levels once the baby is delivered.) When LES pressure is lowered for any reason, it is easier for acid to reflux from the stomach into the esophagus.

So, what causes LES pressures to decrease during pregnancy? First, levels of the hormones estrogen and progesterone are elevated during pregnancy, and elevated levels of these hormones cause the LES pressure to decrease. Second, pressure in the abdominal cavity increases as the uterus enlarges. This pressure may change the anatomy of the gastroesophageal junction in such a way that LES pressure is decreased. Women who are pregnant may also have problems with heartburn because esophageal motility worsens during pregnancy. This means that when acid reflux occurs, the esophagus does not contract as well as it normally does, thereby allowing acid to linger in the esophagus, where it can cause damage.

A woman's description of symptoms is generally sufficient to make a diagnosis of GERD. Symptoms of a burning sensation behind the breastbone with discomfort radiating to the mouth and throat are common. Many women complain of regurgitating fluid or solid food from the stomach into the throat or mouth, especially when they bend over. Some complain of an acid taste or bitter or bile taste in their mouth. Others may have water brash (see Chapter 3). These classic symptoms of acid reflux make the diagnosis fairly certain, and treatment can be started without any diagnostic testing. (By the way, there

are no published studies that show that having heartburn during pregnancy affects the health of the developing fetus in any way.)

Some women who are pregnant may not have classic symptoms,
and their GERD may remain undiagnosed or may be misdiagnosed.
Atypical symptoms of acid reflux disease are the same in pregnant
women as in anyone else, including a change in voice, laryngitis,
asthma, a chronic cough, or chest pain. Many women with these symptoms are given a therapeutic trial of medications to treat presumed acid
reflux disease. If the symptoms clear up on the medication, then the
diagnosis has been confirmed. If the symptoms persist despite treatment, there are several possible explanations. The disease may be severe, requiring more aggressive treatment. Or it may be that the medications are being taken at too low a dose to be effective (a common
occurrence during pregnancy, when most patients and doctors want to
minimize the use of medications), or that the symptoms are not due to
acid reflux after all. When symptoms persist despite adequate treatment, the patient may be referred for diagnostic testing (see Chapter 4).

Most doctors prefer not to perform diagnostic tests on a woman
who is pregnant, but sometimes it is necessary. Of the various tests
used to diagnose GERD, the barium swallow and the upper GI series
are *not* recommended for pregnant women, because of the danger of
radiation exposure for the developing baby. Although a 24-hour pH
probe or esophageal manometry is considered safe, most physicians
also try to wait (if it is safe to do so) to perform these tests until after the
baby is born. Doctors generally try to avoid performing any invasive
tests on pregnant patients unless absolutely necessary.

Upper endoscopy (EGD) during pregnancy deserves special men-
tion. Several scientific studies have demonstrated that this diagnostic
test is safe even during pregnancy. Women who have this test during
pregnancy deliver babies whose weight, Apgar scores (scores that
measure the health status of the child at birth), and overall health are
the same as those of babies whose mothers did not have endoscopy. In
addition, there is no indication that EGD induces premature labor.
Concern has been raised about the safety of this procedure owing to
the need for conscious sedation. (Recall that most patients receive a
narcotic and a sedative during the procedure so that it can be per-

formed safely and painlessly.) Although not directly approved for use by the Food and Drug Administration during pregnancy, the drugs used during EGD appear to be safe for use during pregnancy if given in small amounts and especially if given later in pregnancy, during the second or third trimester.

We recommend that endoscopy be performed in pregnant patients only if there is evidence of bleeding or if the patient has difficulty swallowing, or if heartburn symptoms are so severe that they are disabling, despite the aggressive use of medications. We do not recommend upper endoscopy during the first trimester unless it is an absolute emergency. This is because the fetus is most vulnerable to damage during the first trimester of pregnancy, when vital organ systems (lung, heart, brain) are still developing.

Pregnant women with acid reflux disease must have their disease treated in a way that avoids or at least minimizes the use of any medication that might be absorbed by the developing fetus. The initial therapy for all pregnant women with acid reflux disease should be lifestyle modifications (see Chapter 5). We recommend eating a light evening meal, waiting at least three or four hours between the end of dinner and going to bed, avoiding nighttime snacks, and avoiding fatty foods and greasy foods. It is also very important to avoid alcohol and smoking, not only because they can make heartburn worse but also because they can injure the developing fetus.

The most important lifestyle modification is elevating the head of the bed. This simple step can, by itself, often minimize or even eliminate heartburn. Raising the head of the bed six inches with blocks or bricks elevates the esophagus above the stomach, which makes it much harder for acidic gastric secretions to injure the esophagus. For some pregnant women, elevating the head of the bed six inches is too uncomfortable, interrupts their sleep, or makes them feel as if they were sliding out of bed. Although not as effective as elevating the head of the bed with blocks or bricks, a foam wedge can be placed under the shoulders to elevate the esophagus above the stomach. Using two or three pillows stacked together to elevate the mouth and esophagus above the stomach is another possibility, but it is much less effective than blocks, bricks, or a foam wedge.

If a pregnant woman continues to have heartburn even with life-style modifications, antacids are the next line of therapy (see Chapter 6). Antacids are generally considered safe during pregnancy because with few exceptions they are not well absorbed by the gastrointestinal tract. The one antacid we do *not* recommend using is sodium bicarbonate (baking soda), which has a high sodium content and can cause significant fluid retention, which may already be a problem in pregnancy. If used in large doses, baking soda can also make the blood too alkaline, which can be dangerous.

For women whose reflux symptoms occur primarily in the evening or at bedtime, a dose of antacid at bedtime or a dose after dinner and another at bedtime may be all that is needed. We recommend taking one to two tablespoons of a liquid antacid (Mylanta or Maalox II) one hour after meals and at bedtime. Women who require a second medication in addition to routine doses of liquid antacids often achieve relief by taking alginic acid two to four times a day. Alginic acid (Gaviscon) is thought to float on top of the gastric secretions; when the gastric secretions are washed back up into the esophagus, the alginic acid coats the esophagus and protects it from injury.

Although the over-the-counter dose of any of the H_2-blockers is smaller than a prescription dose, these medications are well absorbed by the body and are passed into the developing fetus or into the nursing child through breast milk. Admittedly, the amount of medication that enters the baby's body will probably be small, as the medication is largely diluted when it is absorbed into the mother's body. Without any good evidence showing that these drugs are safe during pregnancy and breastfeeding, however, we cannot routinely recommend them.

Fortunately, most pregnant women who have acid reflux find that their symptoms respond to lifestyle modifications and liquid antacids or alginic acid. Pregnant women who continue to have significant acid reflux symptoms, however, may need to take prescription-strength medications. Although many medications are safe to take during pregnancy, there is always the concern that the medications will injure the developing fetus, and health care providers try to avoid or minimize the use of any unnecessary medications during pregnancy.

Most women having severe symptoms of GERD will not, during the

FDA Safety Classification of Medications Used during Pregnancy

Class A: Studies in humans have not demonstrated any risk to the fetus. It is recommended, however, that medications in this class be used only if absolutely necessary.

Class B: Studies in humans demonstrate no risk to the fetus, while animal studies show some risk; or, no adequate human studies have been performed, and animal studies do not demonstrate any risk to the fetus.

Class C: No human studies are available, and animal studies demonstrate increased fetal risk; or, there are not any human or animal studies available.

Class D: Experimental studies demonstrate increased risk to the fetus, but the possible benefits of the drug outweigh the risks. Drugs in this class are generally reserved for life-threatening situations or for severe disease against which safe drugs are ineffective.

course of a pregnancy, develop any of the complications described in Chapter 8, even if they do not take GERD medications. Any pregnant woman with severe GERD symptoms should stay in regular contact with her physician, however, so that the physician can closely monitor changes in symptoms that might indicate a complication.

The Food and Drug Administration (the government agency responsible for reviewing all medications and determining their safety and their proper use in different populations) has devised a rating scale to help physicians and patients decide whether a drug is safe to use during pregnancy. Medications are generally rated as Class A, B, C, or D. Class A medications are considered the safest, while a Class D medication is not considered safe for routine use during pregnancy (see box, above). (The safety classification of drugs used during breast-feeding is slightly different. See box, page 145.)

FDA Safety Classification of Drugs Used while Breastfeeding

Group I: Drug does not enter breast milk.

Group II: Drug enters breast milk but is not thought to affect the baby if used in therapeutic doses.

Group IIIA: Not known whether the drug enters breast milk, but no adverse effects are expected.

Group IIIB: Not known whether the drug enters breast milk, but because the drug is systemically absorbed, it is not recommended.

Group IV: The drug enters breast milk and is not recommended.

As discussed in Chapters 6 and 7, H_2-blockers are very safe for the vast majority of patients. However, all H_2-blockers cross the placenta, and thus there is always the potential for these drugs to affect the developing fetus. We seldom recommend any of the H_2-blockers for a woman who is pregnant or breastfeeding, unless absolutely necessary, and only then under careful guidance from a doctor. If H_2-blockers are required during pregnancy, then we generally recommend ranitidine (Zantac). This is categorized as a Class B medication, and most gastroenterologists are comfortable prescribing it during the second and third trimesters for patients who absolutely need it. (Box on page 146 lists the FDA pregnancy and breastfeeding classifications of prescription drugs for treating acid reflux disease.)

Although cimetidine (Tagamet) is also listed as a Class B medication, some studies suggest that cimetidine can cross the placenta and interfere with the effects of a class of sex hormones called androgens. Androgens play a critical role in the sexual development of the fetus, and thus there is concern that chronic exposure of the fetus to cimetidine could alter sexual development. It is important to note that these risks are primarily theoretical, and that there have not been any reports of injury to humans when cimetidine was taken during pregnancy. Bear-

Safety Profile of Prescription Medications Used for Acid Reflux during Pregnancy and while Breastfeeding

Medication	FDA Classification	Breastfeeding Classification
H_2-blockers		
Cimetidine (Tagamet)	Class B	Group IV
Famotidine (Pepcid)	Class B	Group IV
Nizatidine (Axid)	Class C	Group IV
Ranitidine (Zantac)	Class B	Group IV
Proton-pump inhibitors		
Lansoprazole (Prevacid)	Class B	See note, below
Omeprazole (Prilosec)	Class C	"
Pantoprazole (Protonix)	Class B	"
Rabeprazole (Aciphex)	Class B	"
Esomeprazole (Nexium)	Class B	"
Prokinetic agent		
Metoclopramide (Reglan)	Class B	Group IV
Others		
Sucralfate (Carafate)	Class B	Group IIIA
Antacids	Class B	Group II

Note: As a group, all proton-pump inhibitors are expected to enter breast milk, and we do not recommend their use for mothers who breastfeed, as their safety is unknown.

ing that in mind, however, we do not routinely recommend cimetidine during pregnancy.

Finally, among the H_2-blockers, we also do not recommend nizatidine (Axid) during pregnancy. Nizatidine has been categorized as a Class C medication by the FDA because studies have shown that animals treated with nizatidine during pregnancy delivered newborns lower in weight than the newborns of animals not treated with nizatidine. In addition, there were fewer live animals in each litter. Although it is sometimes difficult to extrapolate animal data to everyday clinical practice, in this situation we believe that given the variety of other alternatives, there are no advantages to the use of this medication during pregnancy, and it should therefore be avoided.

What about the proton-pump inhibitors? How safe are they during pregnancy? Omeprazole (Prilosec) has been shown to cross the placenta in sheep, and it is assumed from these studies that it can also cross the placenta in humans. Because of this, omeprazole is labeled by the FDA as a Class C medication, and it should be avoided during pregnancy and while breastfeeding (see box, page 146). Lansoprazole (Prevacid), pantoprazole (Protonix), and rabeprazole (Aciphex) are all classified by the FDA as Class B medications. Esomeprazole (Nexium), recently approved by the FDA for sale in the United States, is also labeled a Class B medication. Although these drugs are given a higher classification by the FDA than omeprazole, and are thus considered safer to use during pregnancy, we recommend that women not take them during pregnancy and while breastfeeding unless absolutely necessary, because there is just not enough evidence to show that they can be safely used in these circumstances.

The Older Patient

Like many other diseases, GERD appears to become more common with increasing age, for a variety of reasons. First, older patients are more likely than younger patients to visit doctors, who may ask them about heartburn symptoms; thus, older patients are more likely to report these symptoms than younger patients. Second, older patients are generally taking more medications than younger patients. As we've learned, some of these medications, such as calcium-channel blockers, theophylline, and nitrates, cause pressure in the lower esophageal sphincter to decrease, which then makes heartburn more likely. Third, esophageal contractions (motility) may decrease with age. This means that any acid that washes back up into the esophagus can linger there and cause problems. Fourth, hiatal hernias are more common in older patients. As discussed in Chapter 2, hiatal hernias can change the anatomy of the gastroesophageal junction and weaken its natural anti-reflux barrier.

Although GERD may be more prevalent in older patients than in younger patients, the symptoms of GERD do not change. Regurgitation, a burning sensation behind the breastbone that radiates to the mouth, water brash (see Chapter 3), or an acid taste in the mouth are all classic symptoms of GERD in the older person. The burning pain behind the breastbone may cause the older patient the most worry, however, because it can easily be confused with the chest pain associated with heart disease.

Diagnostic studies for evaluating the older patient with heartburn symptoms are the same as those described in Chapter 4. There are no limitations based on age for performing an upper endoscopy or a 24-hour pH probe. Most gastroenterologists who perform these tests, however, are more cautious with the older patient. Many older patients are taking multiple medications, which always have the potential to interact with the intravenous medications used during conscious sedation. In addition, older patients are more likely to have active medical problems such as angina or emphysema that could make undergoing any type of invasive procedure, such as upper endoscopy, riskier.

A stepwise approach to treatment is always recommended for older patients, beginning with lifestyle modifications. H_2-blockers can safely be taken by older people, as can proton-pump inhibitors and prokinetics such as metoclopramide. Doctors need to review carefully the medication list of all patients, but they must pay special attention to this matter with older patients. For one thing, this group of patients is more likely to be taking medications that can induce or worsen GERD because of their effects on the LES. In addition, people taking multiple medications are at higher risk of having an adverse drug reaction.

Older patients have more complications of acid reflux disease than younger patients. Chronic acid reflux disease that has been untreated or only partially treated may, over a period of years, produce a stricture of the esophagus and cause difficulty swallowing. Chronic acid reflux disease is also a risk factor for the development of Barrett's esophagus.

(See Chapter 8 for a complete discussion of complications and the treatment of complications.)

The Bed-Bound Patient

People may be confined to bed for any number of reasons, including spinal cord injury, severe cerebral palsy, and stroke. Many bed-bound patients suffer from severe acid reflux disease because they are in bed all or most of the time. One large study recently reported by a research group in the Netherlands, for example, confirmed high levels of acid reflux disease in institutionalized individuals who require full-time care. Many of these patients had evidence of prolonged or persistent acid reflux, including esophagitis, and they had a much higher than normal rate of Barrett's esophagus and esophageal strictures.

Acid reflux occurs for a variety of reasons in people who are mostly bed-bound. First, sometimes such people cannot communicate well and thus cannot inform their friends, family, or caregivers that they are suffering from GERD symptoms. Second, a person who is flat in bed all or most of the day is at a mechanical disadvantage. In this position, the esophagus is often on the same level as the stomach, which makes it easy for acid to wash up into the esophagus. Finally, many such people are taking medications that decrease pressure in the lower esophageal sphincter and make heartburn more likely.

Diagnostic testing and treatment are the same for this group of individuals as for people who are not bed-bound. The first "diagnostic test" in this case, however, requires a high index of suspicion on the part of the health care provider and family members. That is, if there is a reasonable concern that acid reflux is occurring, even if the patient cannot communicate that he or she is having symptoms of acid reflux, then we recommend empiric therapy with a proton-pump inhibitor. Clues that the patient is having acid reflux are water brash (see Chapter 3), excessive salivation, a loss of appetite, a loss of weight, chronic nausea, or coughing or wheezing. We prefer to use the strongest medicine available right from the start for such people, because these medicines usually need to be taken only once a day, they quickly eliminate symptoms, and they rapidly promote healing of the injured esophagus. In addition, if the symptoms clear up after a trial of medication, then the diagnosis of acid reflux disease is confirmed, and no special tests need to be performed. This is important, because many of these tests can be difficult or stressful for patients who are bed-bound.

Lifestyle modifications are also helpful to people who are confined to bed. We usually recommend that they have smaller, more frequent meals or feedings. This helps the stomach empty more efficiently and minimizes the chance that reflux will occur. For patients on a purely liquid diet, the use of commercial thickeners may help reduce the amount of reflux and also minimize the risk of aspiration (food or liquid entering the lungs). We recommend that feedings be performed in an upright position if possible, or at a minimum of a 45-degree angle if the patient cannot sit upright.

For bed-bound patients who have reflux disease, we recommend immediate therapy with H_2-blockers or proton-pump inhibitors rather than beginning therapy with lifestyle modifications and antacids. Many of these patients already have significant medical problems, and a complication of GERD, such as an esophageal stricture, could be life-threatening.

Some patients who are bed-bound or incapacitated develop complications from acid reflux disease before treatment begins. As noted in the Netherlands study, they may develop an esophageal stricture or Barrett's esophagus. Often, the most difficult part of evaluating and treating bed-bound and chronically ill patients is first to consider the diagnosis of acid reflux disease, even if the patient does not complain of typical symptoms. To avoid symptoms and complications, the difficulty of evaluating a bed-bound patient must be overcome to assess and treat GERD appropriately and in a timely way.

In this chapter we have reviewed the particular considerations that must be taken into account in diagnosing and treating GERD in special populations of patients. As in previous chapters, the focus has been on current methods of diagnosis and treatment. In the final section of the book we look into the future, to a time not far from now when, we hope, diagnosing and treating GERD will be more effective and less invasive than ever, for all patients.

Part V

THE FUTURE

Chapter 10

A Look into the Future

Diagnosing and Treating GERD and Complications of GERD

For many years people with GERD were advised by their doctors to avoid spicy foods, eat a bland diet, and minimize stress. Flare-ups of acid reflux were generally treated with liquid antacids—often by the bottleful. We're glad to be able to say that over the past 25 years, dramatic progress has been made in the treatment of acid reflux disease. For one thing, doctors understand much more about what causes GERD, and this understanding helps them give patients specific advice about lifestyle changes that can often eliminate symptoms. In addition, as Chapters 6 and 7 testify, a large variety of medications are now available to improve or eliminate symptoms of acid reflux and prevent complications of GERD.

Even when their patients get well and stay well, however, most physicians are not content with the status quo when it comes to patient care. They wonder how they can take better care of their patients, how they can detect problems earlier, and how they can prevent complications of diseases, including chronic diseases such as diabetes, high blood pressure, and GERD.

Looking into the future, in this chapter we consider new treatments that are being developed—treatments that will be more convenient and effective in treating GERD. In the future we also expect to see new diagnostic tests coming into use, and these tests will be more accurate and more comfortable for patients than those currently being used to diagnose GERD and its complications. Finally, some promising avenues are opening up with regard to preventing complications, which means that fewer people will suffer from the complications of GERD. Of course, our wish is that someday GERD will no longer be an ongoing medical problem but will instead be a condition that can be avoided or quickly cured. Considering the research currently under way, this may not be an overly optimistic wish.

The Future of Medical Therapy

Improvements in Current Medications

Over the years we have made great strides in developing medications for treating acid reflux. We have more potent medications, so patients take fewer pills. And we have medications whose effects last longer, which means that the pills can be taken much less frequently.

Further improvements are on the horizon. Soon, for example, we may have even more potent acid-suppressing medications. This is important, because although the vast majority of patients can control their symptoms with either H_2-blockers or proton-pump inhibitors taken once or twice a day, some patients require very high doses of these acid-suppressing medications and have to take them as often as four times a day.

Many people have trouble remembering to take a pill four times each day, and most people find such frequent dosing inconvenient, as well. For these patients, *compliance* (taking medications at the scheduled times) may be difficult. But if we had an even more concentrated acid-suppressing medication that could be taken just once a day by patients who need it, then compliance would be much easier. Rabeprazole, for example, is a relatively new proton-pump inhibitor that is taken only once daily. Early results show that it works well when taken once a day, even in people with severe symptoms and severe esophagitis. Pantoprazole is another new proton-pump inhibitor, approved by the Food and Drug Administration at the end of 2000, that shows promising results with once-daily dosing. More medications like these will almost certainly become available shortly. Their improved ability to suppress acid means they will do a better job of preventing complications.

Because GERD is a chronic disease, many patients must take medications every day, for years at a time. Ideally, medications would need to be taken only once a week, or even once a month. Such an easy schedule would certainly be more acceptable to the patient and would probably ensure that most patients would be faithful about taking their medication. It doesn't appear that *oral* medications for acid reflux disease will ever be able to be taken on such an infrequent dosing schedule, however. This is because food or medication that is swallowed normally passes through the entire gastrointestinal tract within 36 hours. Materials that are not completely digested or absorbed within 36 hours are eliminated. Thus, even the capsules used in slow-release forms of medication are usually eliminated within 36 hours, along with any remaining medicine. In addition, new cells that produce gastric acid are constantly being made in the stomach, and thus oral medications for GERD usually need to be given at least once a day to inhibit these newly made cells. So there is not much hope that longer-acting oral medications for GERD can be developed.

Medications can be taken in other forms, however, and one of these alternate routes may well be the future of acid suppression. One technological advance that looks promising for GERD therapy is a patch placed on the skin that slowly releases acid-suppressing medications and lasts up to one week. Such a patch would be resistant to water, so bathing or showering would not be a problem. Once-a-week dosing would be easy, safe, and convenient. Moreover, it would likely increase compliance, and this in turn would lead to better health and fewer complications.

Another method of delivering medications slowly over time is by injection, an approach that is surprisingly acceptable to many patients. One of the best examples of a time-release medicine given by injection is the contraceptive agent Depo-Provera, which has been shown to be safe and effective. Many women who use Depo-Provera find that getting a shot every three to four months is much more convenient than taking a daily birth-control pill. It is possible that similar technology could be useful for medications used to treat GERD. Imagine taking a shot every three to four months to prevent heartburn: no more daily medications, no more missed doses, no more running to the pharmacy every month. Not only might this schedule lead to fewer missed doses, but it might also lead to lower costs and fewer complications.

Although our discussion so far has focused on medications requiring a prescription, changes are also occurring in medications available without a prescription. Many people with occasional symptoms of heartburn initially respond well to an over-the-counter medication, like Tums or Rolaids, that can be chewed and swallowed. Unfortunately, for many people symptoms return one to two hours later. One design for prolonging the relief of symptoms is to combine a chewable antacid with an H_2-blocker. This combination would provide immediate relief via the antacid and would also provide relief for the next few hours as the H_2-blocker worked to decrease the production of stomach acid.

Finally, one significant improvement we expect to see over the next few years in regard to both H_2-blockers and proton-pump inhibitors has nothing to do with the effectiveness of the medications. This improvement will be in the *cost* of the medications. When these classes of medications were first developed and released, they were covered by a patent from the company that developed the drug. Drug patents generally last 17 years and are designed to prevent other companies from copying the formula and then releasing their own version, usually at a significantly lower cost. (This 17-year period allows the company that designed the drug to recover its costs for research and development.) In the next few years several of the prescription-strength H_2-blockers and proton-pump inhibitors will no longer be covered by their original patents. This means that other companies can produce the same medication and sell it, and this increased competition translates into cost savings for patients. This will be good news for all patients, because many of these medications are currently very expensive.

New Medications on the Horizon

As we discussed in Chapter 7, one type of medication commonly used to treat GERD is the class of prokinetic agents. Unlike the H_2-blockers and the proton-pump inhibitors, these medications don't block the production of stomach acid. Instead, they increase esophageal motility, the series of coordinated muscular contractions that empty food and liquid out of the esophagus and into the stomach. Prokinetic agents also stimulate gastric emptying. Both of these actions help to decrease the amount of time that acid stays in contact with the lining of the esophagus.

In the next decade there will probably be two significant advances in this type of drug. First, a longer-acting form of the medication is likely to be developed. This will resolve a major shortcoming of these agents. In Chapter 7 we mentioned cisapride, the prokinetic drug that was taken off the market because of the potential for serious side effects in some patients. Several studies demonstrated that cisapride was very effective in treating GERD, either in combination with an H_2-blocker or a proton-pump inhibitor or used alone. One disadvantage of this drug (in addition to the potential for serious side effects) was that it had a short *half-life*, meaning that, once absorbed into the body, it was rapidly broken down and then eliminated. Thus, a single dose worked only for several hours. Most patients who benefited from this drug usually had to take it three or four times a day—before each meal and often also at bedtime—whereas the ideal medication for improved emptying of the esophagus would be taken upon awakening in the morning and then last 14 to 16 hours. This would provide protection all day long, especially after meals. A patient with significant nighttime heartburn could take an additional pill at night. Thus, once-a-day dosing would increase compliance and lead to an improvement in overall health and comfort, and it might also decrease the risk of developing complications from GERD.

The other potential advance in prokinetic agents would be a medication that specifically targeted the lower esophageal sphincter. As

noted in Chapter 2, the LES spends most of its time in a closed position, meaning that stomach acid cannot reflux up into the esophagus.
If this muscle is weak, however, it remains open for longer periods of
time than normal and allows reflux to occur. One medication currently available, metoclopramide, acts to increase the muscular tone of
the LES, but it also affects other sites in the gastrointestinal tract. Medications designed to act specifically and only at the gastroesophageal
junction would dramatically improve symptoms of acid reflux. A
stronger LES, one that spends nearly all of its time contracted rather
than relaxed, would decrease the frequency of acid reflux and also
decrease the length of each episode of acid reflux. Ideally this medication would be taken once a day, or perhaps it could be administered
through a patch or by injection, which would make it easier to take.
Researchers in Australia recently demonstrated that baclofen, a medication that until now was generally used to treat muscle spasms, actually increases pressure in the LES and reduces the number of episodes
of acid reflux. So it is possible that some medications we already use for
other reasons could turn out to be useful in treating GERD.

Two ways to help prevent caustic stomach acid from injuring the
esophagus are, first, minimizing the amount of gastric acid produced
and, second, preventing acid from reaching, or remaining in, the
esophagus. Despite advances in both suppressing acid and improving
LES tone and function, however, some acid may still reflux into the
esophagus and injure it. Because of this, a third approach to protecting
the esophagus from acidic stomach contents is needed: coating the
esophagus with a physical barrier. A medication to coat the esophagus
might come in a chewable pill form or in a liquid form. The active
material would bind to the cells that line the esophagus and form a
protective coating. This thin layer of protective material would not
interfere with the movement of food or liquids into the stomach. If the
material adhered tenaciously to the lining cells of the esophagus, the
medication might have to be taken only once a week or so.

Medicines that function in a similar manner are now available to
help protect the stomach from damage due to aspirin, and to help protect teeth and prevent cavities. Alginic acid has some of these properties: it is washed back into the esophagus from the stomach and pro-

tects the esophagus from caustic stomach acid. But alginic acid does not *bind* to the mucosa (lining cells) of the esophagus; it floats above the surface of the mucosa. This means that the medication is effective only for minutes to hours, rather than days. The ideal esophageal protective medication would actually bind to the cells lining the esophagus and form a long-lasting coating.

The Future of Surgical Therapy

At this time, Nissen fundoplication (described in Chapter 7) is the most effective surgery for treating GERD in people whose symptoms do not respond to medications. The procedure is now performed laparoscopically and is considered relatively safe as well as effective.

The question is whether this operation can be further improved. The fact is that there is room for improvement in almost any type of procedure—improvement that leads to less time in the operating room, shorter hospital stays, and a further decline in the rate of postoperative complications. These are small advances, however; we don't expect any great change in Nissen fundoplication in the next decade or so. There may, in fact, soon be a revolution in acid reflux surgery, but it won't come from the surgeons; it will come from the endoscopists and gastroenterologists.

A new therapeutic option for controlling acid reflux is currently under development. The goal of this new technique is identical to the goal of current surgery for acid reflux disease: to tighten the lower esophageal sphincter so that acid cannot reflux up into the esophagus. What is different about it is that it can be performed during endoscopy and does not require invasive open surgery or laparoscopic surgery with general anesthesia. This new technique is called *endoscopic suturing*. During this procedure, several stitches are placed in the lower esophagus at the level of the LES. These stitches tighten or "cinch up" the lower esophagus. The result is a tighter LES, which in theory will prevent recurrent episodes of acid reflux. Ideally, this would allow patients to remain free of symptoms from acid reflux and also allow them to stop taking acid-suppressing medications.

Preliminary results in a small group of patients in Europe who underwent endoscopic suturing look promising. Patients report both fewer episodes of reflux and a reduction in the use of medications. This technique is now being tested and used in the United States and was approved by the FDA in April 2000. The advantages over surgery include the shorter time of the procedure, the use of conscious sedation rather than general anesthesia, faster recovery time, the elimination of an overnight hospital stay, and lower costs (endoscopic suturing is estimated to cost $3,000 per patient, compared with between $10,000 and $15,000 per patient for Nissen fundoplication). In addition, endoscopic suturing should not prevent, or make difficult, any formal antireflux surgery that might become necessary in the future. Possible disadvantages include internal injury to the esophagus, which could result in bleeding, infection, the development of a stricture, or injury to the nerves of the esophagus or stomach. It is not yet known how these benefits and risks compare with antireflux surgery. In the years to come a direct comparison using large groups of patients will be done to determine which procedure is most effective in both the short run and the long run, and which procedure is most cost-effective.

Another new and lower-cost alternative to antireflux surgery is a technique called the *Stretta procedure.* Like endoscopic suturing, this procedure is performed endoscopically and does not require surgery. During routine upper endoscopy, a special probe is passed into the lower esophagus at the level of the gastroesophageal junction. A balloon is inflated to hold the probe in place and to force specially designed radio-frequency electrodes directly against the mucosa of the esophagus. An electrical current then passes through the radio-frequency electrodes to produce *thermal injury* to the mucosa. This thermal injury amounts to a controlled burn to the mucosa and underlying tissue of the lower esophagus. As the burn heals, it forms scar tissue at the level of the gastroesophageal junction. The scar tissue acts as a physical barrier to prevent reflux of acid from the stomach into the esophagus, thereby relieving symptoms of heartburn.

Initial results from a small number of patients who have undergone the Stretta procedure look promising. But because this procedure was approved by the FDA only in April 2000, no large studies have been done to look at its long-term effectiveness, or to determine whether there are any long-term complications associated with it. The Stretta procedure appears to have great potential, but further studies must be done before it can routinely be recommended to the general public as a safe alternative to the long-term use of medications or to antireflux surgery.

The Future of Diagnosing GERD

In many patients, the diagnosis of GERD is straightforward. If the classic symptoms of GERD (described in Chapter 3) are relieved by antacids or by H_2-blockers or proton-pump inhibitors, then the diagnosis is essentially confirmed, and no further testing is generally required. For patients with uncommon symptoms of GERD, or those who appear to have GERD but fail to respond to therapy, various diagnostic tests (described in Chapter 4) can confirm a diagnosis of GERD or reveal what else is causing the symptoms. In the future, however, advances in the diagnosis of GERD will likely arrive on a number of different fronts.

Upper endoscopy, which allows direct inspection of the lining of the esophagus, can be uncomfortable or unpleasant. Some patients dislike it because of the need for sedation, or the unpleasant taste of the topical anesthetic agents used, or the thickness of the endoscope that passes through the mouth into the esophagus. One improvement in this procedure, and thus in the diagnosis of GERD, will be miniaturization of the endoscope. Technological advances in the electronics industry have made it possible to miniaturize such products as radios, computers, telephones, and cameras, and this process can be applied to the endoscope, and thus endoscopy, as well.

The endoscopes in use today are about as big around as a finger. Now imagine an endoscope with a diameter smaller than that of a pencil. It would be very soft, and very flexible—almost like a piece of cooked pasta. The size of the tube would make it easy to swallow, making the procedure so much more comfortable that intravenous sedation would not be needed. This, in turn, would lead to a significant decrease in the cost of the procedure, which would make it possible for more patients to have the test done. Moreover, the small size of the endoscope, and the ability to use it without sedation, would allow endoscopy to become an office-based procedure, which would allow more rapid identification of those who might need aggressive medical therapy, those at higher risk of developing complications, and those who already have Barrett's esophagus. We expect this type of endoscope—an ultrathin endoscope—to become widely available over the next few years and to be in routine use within the next 10 years.

Disorders of the lower esophageal sphincter are now routinely identified by esophageal manometry. This is a fairly simple test usually taking about one hour. During the test, a thin, flexible tube is passed through the nose into the stomach. Although this test is often very important for diagnostic purposes, some patients cannot tolerate it at all. In the years to come, our ability to measure LES function (and dysfunction) may improve in two different ways. First, if the tube becomes smaller in size, the current procedure may become much more tolerable to some patients. A thinner, more flexible tube would slip into the esophagus more easily. The other improvement in the measurement of LES function may arrive in the form of noninvasive measurements of esophageal function. Most patients, if given a choice, prefer noninvasive testing. Technology has made great strides in the use of radiological imaging techniques such as CT scan (computer tomography scanning) and MRI (magnetic resonance imaging). Rapid sequence scanning of the esophagus with either CT scan or MRI would provide minutely detailed three-dimensional images of the lower esophagus and the lower esophageal sphincter—the area so critical to the development of GERD. One drawback of this technique would be the inability to measure pressures in the LES directly.

Many patients with atypical symptoms of acid reflux disease undergo a 24-hour pH probe. During this test a thin, flexible tube is passed through the nose and into the esophagus, where it remains for 24 hours, measuring changes in the pH of the esophagus to determine when and how often the esophagus is exposed to acidic gastric juices. This test can be important for patients who are considering having surgery to treat chronic acid reflux disease, but many people find it inconvenient or unpleasant. We expect that there will be two improvements in this test in the years to come. First, as with other technologies, the tube will undergo miniaturization and become much thinner, thereby making the procedure more comfortable. Second, although the current scientific thinking is that 24 hours is the ideal duration for this test, advances in data analysis may shorten the time required for a satisfactory test to be performed. Once researchers review the data from tens of thousands of patients, they may find that enough data are obtained during an 8-hour or a 12-hour study to allow decisions to be made regarding changes in medical therapy or the need for surgery. This would eliminate the need for the full 24-hour test. Alternatively, the test may be improved by the addition of various conditions or medications that provoke or "challenge" the competency of the LES and try to provoke acid reflux. If conditions can be employed that maximize the potential for reflux to occur, then the test most likely can be shortened, because useful observations can be made without waiting for them to happen "naturally."

One final improvement that will occur over the next few years in the diagnosis of GERD involves the use of medications. Future research will most likely show that one of the best tests to confirm the diagnosis of GERD in patients with less common symptoms, such as a change in voice or a cough that occurs only at night, is to give them potent acid-suppressing medications, possibly coupled with the use of prokinetic agents. Many patients with these atypical symptoms have normal upper endoscopies and normal upper GI series, and thus their symptoms may not even be considered signs of acid reflux disease, even after diagnostic testing. However, if all symptoms resolve with a two- to four-week trial of potent acid suppression provided by a proton-pump inhibitor, possibly coupled with a prokinetic agent to improve the motility of the esophagus, then the diagnosis is all but confirmed. Because these medicines act only on the gastrointestinal tract, a cough due to an infection or to allergies won't respond to these GI medications and confuse the issue, while a cough due to chronic acid reflux should respond to the trial of medications. Although these medications are sometimes expensive, the aggressive use of potent medications may actually turn out to be not only the *best* initial test to confirm GERD in atypical patients but the most *cost-effective* test as well.

The Future of Diagnosing and Treating the Complications of GERD

Diagnosing Complications

One of the greatest concerns to patients who have had gastroesophageal reflux disease for many years, and for their doctors, is the possibility of Barrett's esophagus. As discussed in Chapter 8, Barrett's esophagus is a premalignant condition of the esophagus, which means that the tissue, although not initially cancerous, has an increased likelihood of developing into esophageal cancer over time. One of the current dilemmas in gastroenterology is determining which patients with GERD should have routine upper endoscopies to look for Barrett's, and how often these routine EGDs should be performed.

Although safe, EGD remains fairly expensive, requires the use of intravenous sedation, and is uncomfortable or unpleasant for some patients. What is needed is a safe, inexpensive, noninvasive test that accurately determines whether a patient has Barrett's esophagus. Such a test would allow the doctor to determine who needs aggressive surveillance so that this premalignant condition can be identified before problems develop.

One answer might be a simple blood test, similar to the prostate-specific antigen (PSA) test, which is now widely used to identify patients with suspected prostate cancer. PSA (a protein that can be detected by an antibody) is released from the prostate gland and travels through the bloodstream and can therefore be measured by a simple blood test. Elevated levels of PSA in the blood do not always mean that the patient has prostate cancer; what it means is that the prostate may be enlarged or infected, or that early cancer may be present. And elevated levels mean that the patient will be evaluated more closely and carefully and that further tests or examinations might be scheduled.

As noted in Chapter 8, in Barrett's esophagus, the normal lining cells of the esophagus (squamous epithelium) are transformed into a different cell type (intestinal-type, columnar epithelium). It is possible that these cells change in other ways as well, producing different proteins or chemicals in response to the cellular transformation. If these chemicals or proteins are released into the blood, then theoretically they could be identified by a blood sample. Thus, a patient with GERD could have a simple blood test to determine if Barrett's esophagus is developing.

In a similar manner, a simple blood test to detect early cancer of the esophagus could also become available. One of the most disturbing characteristics of esophageal cancer is that it can develop in the setting of Barrett's esophagus and grow significantly in size without causing symptoms. Most people with esophageal cancer don't develop any symptoms, such as trouble swallowing, until the cancer has already grown and spread throughout the esophagus and into other parts of the body. By this time it is often not possible to cure it. There are now blood tests available that can be used to help identify certain types of cancer, such as colon cancer (CEA test), prostate cancer (PSA; see above), and cervical cancer (CA 19-9). These blood tests are accurate in some patients, but not in all. For example, these blood tests are elevated in some people who don't have cancer, and normal in some patients who do have cancer. Clearly, there are limits to our present technology. However, many types of cancer cells, including esophageal cancer, produce special proteins or chemicals that are specific to that type of cancer. As the cancer cells begin to grow and spread, they often release these chemicals into the bloodstream. If chemicals or proteins unique to early esophageal cancer could be identified in the blood, then we might have an early-warning system for patients at risk of developing invasive esophageal cancer.

At the present time, the only way to diagnose Barrett's esophagus with certainty is to perform an EGD and take samples of tissue that looks suspicious. Barrett's esophagus usually looks different from the surrounding normal esophageal tissue, but in some patients it is hard for the endoscopist to observe the slight difference in color between normal tissue and Barrett's tissue. In addition, some patients have only a very short segment of Barrett's (less than half an inch long), and this can be very difficult to spot. Over the last few years several researchers have developed dyes that seem to bind only to Barrett's tissue and not to normal tissue. At the time of endoscopy these dyes can be sprayed through the endoscope and onto the lower esophagus. If the patient has Barrett's, then the dye attaches to that tissue, which helps to highlight it and make it easier to see. The endoscopist can then take biopsies of this highlighted area to verify the diagnosis of Barrett's esophagus. Although still in the early stages, this technique looks very promising, especially as a means of detecting Barrett's in patients with very short segments of this abnormal tissue.

However promising, this new technique for diagnosing Barrett's esophagus still depends on the taking of samples of tissue during an EGD. Some patients don't want to have this test because it can be uncomfortable or because it requires sedation. And some patients can't afford the test. So, can samples of tissue be obtained without endoscopy? The answer is yes, but not yet in the United States. In some parts of Asia the risk of cancer of the stomach and esophagus is much higher than it is in the United States. In these areas of Asia, health care workers attempt to routinely evaluate and screen patients for these cancers. Performing EGDs on millions of patients for screening purposes would be prohibitively expensive, so researchers have developed a device that looks somewhat like a balloon attached to the end of a soft, flexible tube. The balloon, which has bumps and ridges on it, is passed through the mouth into the esophagus or stomach. It is then inflated and moved back and forth. The raised areas on the balloon rub against the lining of the esophagus or stomach and pick up cells. The balloon is then deflated and withdrawn, and the cells are collected from the surface of the balloon and evaluated for evidence of early cancer.

The advantages of this test are many. It is safe, does not require sedation, can be performed in the office, and is very inexpensive. In addition, unlike blood tests, it retrieves cells that can be directly examined for the changes that occur in cancer. There are some disadvantages, however. Some patients cannot tolerate the balloon or the procedure without sedation, and thus would be excluded from this screening test. In addition, the balloon does not always reliably collect cells, and in those cases there is nothing to examine under the microscope. Finally, the balloon cannot be used to biopsy a specific area of tissue. Thus, a person could have an area of Barrett's, but if the balloon did not come into contact with that area, then the report would falsely conclude that Barrett's was not present. This test holds promise for a safe, easy method to identify patients with Barrett's esophagus, but further work needs to be done before it can be recommended to the U.S. public.

Treating Complications

When Barrett's esophagus is identified on EGD, the first step in any treatment regimen is to prevent further injury to the lower esophagus, if possible, usually through the use of a proton-pump inhibitor once or twice a day to suppress acid. The next step is to remove the premalignant tissue. The theory is that removal of the Barrett's tissue will allow normal, healthy tissue to develop in its place. It can be very difficult to remove the tissue, however. In addition, even if the Barrett's tissue is removed, there is no guarantee that only normal, healthy tissue will grow in its place. In some cases Barrett's tissue grows instead of normal tissue.

Small areas of Barrett's can be burned away using an electrical cautery device during EGD. This technique is usually not used for large areas, however, as it may result in perforation (a hole or tear) of the esophagus or the development of a stricture. How, then, can these segments of Barrett's be eliminated?

One technique currently being investigated at Johns Hopkins uses liquid nitrogen to freeze the tissue. This technique has been used in the past to remove skin lesions such as warts. Liquid nitrogen is applied directly to the skin growth, which then freezes. Over the next 7 to 10 days the tissue dries up and falls off. Preliminary results have shown that this technique can remove Barrett's tissue safely. Risks of this procedure include prolonged exposure to the liquid nitrogen, which could permanently damage the esophagus. And once again, there is no guarantee that only healthy tissue will grow back in the area where Barrett's was removed. For people with Barrett's esophagus, however, this technique holds considerable promise.

A novel technique to eliminate segments of Barrett's was developed several years ago and is now being used at several research centers throughout the country. It involves the intravenous infusion of a chemical that is taken up inside of cells—all cells—throughout the body. When exposed to light, the chemical has a chemical reaction with oxygen. This reaction kills the cells that absorbed the chemical. Patients with Barrett's esophagus receive an intravenous injection of the chemical and then 48 hours later undergo EGD. During this procedure a special light is inserted through the endoscope into the esophagus. The light shines on the Barrett's cells, and activates the chemical inside the cells. A chemical reaction occurs, and the cells die. The advantage of this procedure is that it can be used to eliminate large areas of Barrett's esophagus safely. The risks of perforation are very low. Preliminary data from research centers that use this technique, called *photodynamic therapy* (PDT), look very good. Even early esophageal cancers have been eliminated using this technique.

The obvious disadvantage to photodynamic therapy is that *all* cells absorb the chemical and thus potentially can be injured by light, if it is intense enough. Because sunlight is strong enough to initiate the chemical reaction, patients are instructed to cover all exposed areas of their skin for four to six weeks after receiving the chemical, to avoid injury to their skin. A person who lives in a very sunny area, such as Florida, Arizona, or California, can find it difficult to stay out of the sun for such a long period.

Another therapy currently under investigation to treat Barrett's esophagus involves physically stripping the lining tissue away during endoscopy. Again, the theory is that removing the segment of Barrett's esophagus will eliminate the risk of developing cancer of the esophagus because normal cells will grow back in place of the abnormal cells. This treatment requires an EGD as well. During this procedure, sterile saline (saltwater) is injected just under the surface of the Barrett's epithelium. The Barrett's is then physically torn off, leaving tissue underneath that will heal and (again, theoretically) replace the removed tissue with normal tissue. This technique is still in its infancy, and concern exists about whether it can be safely used to remove large segments of Barrett's.

Finally, a new technique called *argon plasma coagulation* (APC) has been developed over the past few years and is now being tested at several research and academic centers throughout the United States, Europe, and Asia. It is similar to the electrical cauterization used to remove small segments of Barrett's tissue, described above, and it, too, requires an EGD. During therapy, a beam of argon is ejected from a special catheter, or tube, and the argon is then immediately ignited by a spark to produce a miniature flame. Argon plasma coagulation can be used to remove large segments of Barrett's because unlike electrical cauterization, it burns only the surface of the esophagus and, in theory, cannot burn all the way through the esophagus. Possible complications include bleeding (uncommon) and the formation of a stricture. Patients with large areas of Barrett's may need several treatments. This may become one of the most effective ways to eliminate large areas of Barrett's, although direct comparisons with the other techniques described above are needed to determine which techniques are safest and provide the best results.

Over the last 25 years, great strides have been made in the diagnosis and treatment of GERD as well as in preventing and treating complications of GERD. Although GERD and its complications are still a problem for many people, we believe that significant and dramatic progress will continue to be made in these areas during the next few years.

In closing, we want to emphasize the importance of educating yourself about GERD. There is so much that can be done today, both to relieve symptoms and to avoid complications. Use this book as a checklist for your own situation, and then be sure to talk things over with your physician or other health care provider. We hope this book will provide both education and reassurance, and that it will encourage people to take action to improve their health.

Abbreviations

APC	argon plasma coagulation
CEA	carcinoembryonic antigen
CT	computed tomography (also called CAT scan, for computer-assisted tomography)
EGD	esophagogastroduodenoscopy
ENT	ear, nose, and throat
FDA	Food and Drug Administration
GE	gastroesophageal
GERD	gastroesophageal reflux disease
GI	gastrointestinal
H_2	histamine receptor type 2
i.v.	intravenous
LES	lower esophageal sphincter
MRI	magnetic resonance imaging
OTC	over-the-counter
PDT	photodynamic therapy
PSA	prostate-specific antigen

Glossary

abdomen The area between the chest and the hips. Contains the stomach, small intestine, large intestine, liver, gallbladder, pancreas, and spleen.

acid reflux The movement of caustic gastric acid from the stomach into the esophagus.

acute A term used to identify a disorder, disease, or process that is sudden in onset and often severe but lasts only a short time.

alimentary canal *See* **gastrointestinal tract.**

anemia A low blood count as measured by hemoglobin or hematocrit.

antacids Medicines that are used to neutralize acidic conditions in the stomach and esophagus.

barium A radio-opaque substance used to coat the inside of a hollow organ such as the esophagus or stomach so that it can be visualized on an x-ray. A radio-opaque substance is one that x-rays do not penetrate well, so that it shows up on an x-ray as a white area.

barium swallow An x-ray test in which a patient swallows barium (see above), which then coats the esophagus so that abnormalities in the esophagus can be identified.

Barrett's esophagus A condition wherein the normal lining cells of the lower esophagus have been replaced by a different, stomach-like cell type owing to repeated irritation and inflammation from stomach acid that has refluxed into the lower esophagus. This change in the cell type, called intestinal metaplasia, has the potential to turn into esophageal cancer in some patients.

biopsy The technique whereby a small piece of tissue is removed from an organ or structure so that it can be examined underneath the microscope. During upper endoscopy, a biopsy may be taken of your stomach or of your lower esophagus.

bougienage The French term for dilation of the esophagus using rubber tubes or other dilators.

CA 19-9 A protein in the blood that can be measured and used as a potential marker for cancer of the cervix.

CEA Carcinoembryonic antigen. A protein in the blood that is sometimes used as a marker for the presence of cancer of the colon or rectum.

chronic A term used to identify a disorder, disease, or process that continues for a long time or recurs frequently.

coagulation Heating of tissue. The extreme heat causes the cells to die. This technique can also be used to seal blood vessels that are leaking and to burn off unwanted tissue.

conscious sedation The technique of using intravenous medications to make the patient feel comfortable and relaxed during a procedure such as upper endoscopy but not to induce sleep.

diaphragm The muscle between the chest and the abdomen. It is the major muscle that the body uses for breathing.

digestion The process the body uses to break down food into simple substances for energy, growth, and cell repair.

digestive system The organs in the body that break down and absorb food. Organs that make up the digestive tract (gastrointestinal tract) are the mouth, esophagus, stomach, small intestine, large intestine, rectum, and anus. Organs that help with digestion but are not part of the digestive tract are the tongue, salivary glands in the mouth, pancreas, liver, and gallbladder.

digestive tract *See* **gastrointestinal tract.**

dilation A procedure designed to stretch a narrowed portion of the esophagus.

duodenum The first part of the small intestine. It is connected to the stomach by a circular muscle called the pylorus.

dysphagia Difficulty swallowing. This may occur because of severe heartburn, the presence of a stricture (narrowing) of the esophagus, or even cancer of the esophagus.

endoscope A flexible, lighted tube with a lens on the end. It is designed to look into your stomach and esophagus (upper endoscopy) or your colon (colonoscopy).

endoscopic suturing A new technique used to treat acid reflux disease. Approved by the Food and Drug Administration in April 2000. Sutures are placed in the lower esophagus to plicate (tighten) it. This has been shown to improve symptoms of acid reflux disease and may be an alternative to anti-reflux surgery.

endoscopist A medical or surgical doctor who uses an endoscope to view the interior of bodily organs like the stomach.

endoscopy A procedure that uses an endoscope to diagnose or treat a condition.

erosion An open sore or break in the lining (the mucosa) of the esophagus or stomach. Commonly caused by gastric acid.

esophageal manometry A test that uses a soft, flexible tube to measure the strength and pressure of the esophagus and the esophageal sphincters.

esophageal reflux *See* **gastroesophageal reflux disease (GERD).**

esophageal stricture A narrowing of the esophagus often caused by acid flowing back from the stomach. A stricture is usually treated by dilating the esophagus, although it occasionally requires surgery.

esophagitis Irritation and inflammation of the esophagus, usually caused by acid that flows up from the stomach.

esophagogastroduodenoscopy (EGD) A procedure that uses an endoscope to look into the esophagus, stomach, and upper small intestine (duodenum). Also called upper endoscopy.

esophagus The muscular tube that connects the mouth to the stomach. Approximately 10 inches long.

fundus The top part of the stomach.

gastric Related to the stomach.

gastric juices Liquids produced in the stomach to help break down food and kill bacteria.

gastroenterologist A doctor who specializes in diagnosing and treating diseases of the digestive system.

gastroenterology The field of medicine concerned with the structure and function of the digestive system.

gastroesophageal reflux disease (GERD) The movement of caustic gastric juices from the stomach back up into the esophagus for an abnormally large amount of time. This movement usually occurs as a result of weakness in the lower esophageal sphincter. Prolonged episodes of reflux may cause esophagitis, esophageal erosions or ulcers, esophageal strictures, Barrett's esophagus, and even cancer of the esophagus. GERD is also called esophageal reflux or reflux esophagitis.

gastrointestinal tract The large, muscular tube that extends from the mouth to the anus. It includes the mouth, esophagus, stomach, small intestine, large intestine, rectum, and anus. Also called the alimentary tract or digestive tract.

heartburn A burning sensation caused by stomach acid after it moves into the lower esophagus and irritates the lining of the esophagus. It is usually felt in the upper abdomen, in the lower chest, or behind the breastbone (sternum).

Helicobacter pylori A curved bacterium that, when present, may cause an ulcer in the stomach or duodenum. This bacterium does not play a significant role in acid reflux disease.

H₂-blockers Also called H_2 receptor antagonists, or H_2 RAs. A class of medications that act on the cells in the stomach responsible for producing and secreting hydrochloric acid. As a group, these medicines act on the histamine type-2 receptor found in acid-secreting cells. There are four medications in this category of drug: cimetidine, famotidine, nizatidine, and ranitidine.

hydrochloric acid An acid made in the stomach. Hydrochloric acid works with pepsin and other enzymes to break down protein in food. It is one of the agents responsible for the damage caused to the esophagus when reflux occurs.

intestinal metaplasia A process that occurs in the esophagus whereby the normal lining cells of the lower esophagus (squamous epithelium) are transformed into a new type of tissue (intestinal-type epithelium) as a result of repeated inflammation and irritation from acid reflux. *See also* **Barrett's esophagus.**

lower esophageal sphincter (LES) A circular muscle, approximately one and one-half inches in length, located at the junction of the esophagus and the stomach. When contracted, it prevents stomach acid from refluxing up into the esophagus. If it relaxes too frequently, or for prolonged periods of time, then gastric acid can easily rush up into the esophagus and cause heartburn.

motility The normal process, coordinated by nerves and smooth muscle, that results in coordinated contractions. In the digestive tract, motility results in the movement of food and products of food digestion through the GI tract.

mucosa The cells that join together to form an inner lining for the different areas of the intestinal tract. The mucosa helps to protect the cells underneath from caustic agents or harmful products. The mucosa of the esophagus is made up of one cell type called squamous epithelium, while the mucosa of the stomach is made up of another cell type called columnar epithelium.

mucus A clear liquid made by cells that line the intestinal tract. Mucus coats and protects tissues in the gastrointestinal tract.

Nissen fundoplication A surgical procedure wherein the upper part of the stomach (the fundus) is wrapped around the lower part of the esophagus. This is performed to help tighten the lower esophageal sphincter and to prevent or minimize acid reflux.

pepsin An enzyme made in the stomach that breaks down proteins. May be partially responsible for damage to the esophagus when reflux of gastric contents occurs.

peptic ulcer A sore in the lining of the stomach or duodenum. This may develop because of excess stomach acid, the use of aspirin, the use of anti-inflammatory agents, or the presence of a bacterium called *Helicobacter pylori*.

perforation A hole that develops in a hollow organ like the esophagus or the stomach. A perforation may be the result of acid causing a large ulcer that then breaks open, or it may be due to trauma caused by a foreign object in the esophagus or stomach (a sharp piece of glass, a large bone accidentally swallowed, an endoscope).

peristalsis The muscular contractions of the gastrointestinal tract that move materials from the mouth to the anus.

pH A measure of how acidic (pH less than 7.0) or how alkaline (basic; pH greater than 7.0) a solution is. Water is used as the standard and has a pH of 7.0.

pharynx The space behind the mouth. It serves as a passageway for food from the mouth to the esophagus and for air from the nose and mouth to the larynx and then into the lungs.

prokinetic agents A group of medications that act on the esophagus and/or stomach to increase contractions in these organs. They help to empty the esophagus and stomach of retained food or secretions, like stomach acid. Metoclopramide (Reglan) is a commonly prescribed prokinetic agent.

proton-pump inhibitors A class of medications that act on the cells in the stomach that produce and secrete hydrochloric acid. At present, these are the most potent acid-suppressing medications we have available. There are currently five types of proton-pump inhibitors available in the United States: lansoprazole, pantoprazole, omeprazole, rabeprazole, and esomeprazole.

PSA Prostate-specific antigen. A protein in the blood that can be measured by a blood test. Often used as a marker for prostate cancer.

pylorus The circular muscle at the junction of the stomach and duodenum. When contracted (closed), it prevents gastric contents from leaving the stomach and entering the duodenum.

pyrosis The burning sensation in the upper abdomen or lower chest due to acid reflux disease. More commonly referred to as heartburn.

reflux *See* **acid reflux.**

reflux esophagitis Irritation and inflammation of the esophagus due to the movement of gastric contents up into the esophagus.

regurgitation The unexpected, involuntary movement of fluids or solids from the stomach into the esophagus or mouth.

saliva A mixture of water, protein, salts, and bicarbonate that makes food easy to swallow, begins the process of digestion, and helps protect the esophagus from stomach acid.

stomach The J-shaped muscular organ designed to hold food, mix and grind food, and empty the ground-up food into the small intestine. The stomach also produces a variety of chemicals, the most important of which is hydrochloric acid. This is the acid responsible for causing heartburn when it refluxes into the lower esophagus.

Stretta procedure A new procedure to help prevent acid reflux disease. Approved by the Food and Drug Administration in April 2000. This procedure uses radio-frequency electrodes to heat the lower esophagus and produce a thermal burn. This later causes the formation of scar tissue, which acts to prevent acid reflux.

stricture A narrowing of a hollow organ due to a congenital condition, trauma, poor blood flow, or inflammation. In the esophagus, strictures can develop because of repeated injury by gastric acid that refluxes up into the lower esophagus. Strictures are usually first noticed by the patient when they cause difficulty swallowing (dysphagia).

24-hour pH probe A test that measures the amount of acid present in the esophagus over a 24-hour period.

ulcer A sore on the lining of the esophagus, stomach, or intestine. Often caused by excess acid, various medications, poor blood flow, or the bacterium *Helicobacter pylori.*

upper endoscopy *See* **esophagogastroduodenoscopy.**

upper esophageal sphincter The circular band of muscles at the top of the esophagus. It is usually contracted and helps to prevents acid from moving from the esophagus into the lungs and mouth.

upper GI series Upper gastrointestinal series. An x-ray study that usually employs barium as the contrast agent. A patient will swallow the barium, which then coats the esophagus, the stomach, and the upper small intestine. X-rays are then taken to look for abnormalities in the lining of these organs, such as ulcers, erosions, strictures, or cancer.

water brash The accumulation of foamy or frothy secretions in the mouth in response to acid reflux. These secretions are produced by the salivary glands and are rich in sodium bicarbonate, which can neutralize gastric acid.

Where to Go for Further Information & Support

www.acg.gi.org/acg-dev/patientinfo/frame--gerd.htm
  "Understanding GERD." A web site maintained by the American College of Gastroenterology, a national organization representing a large number of gastroenterologists. The information on this web site is straightforward, unbiased, and up-to-date. The ACG can be contacted at 4900 B South 31st St., Arlington, VA 22206; 703-820-7400.

www.pharminfo.com/disease/gerd/gerd—infor.html
  "Heartburn/GERD Information Center." A web site maintained by the pharmaceutical industry. It presents general information on GERD and primarily focuses on medications used to treat it.

www.gerd.com/
  "GERD Information Resource Center." A web site maintained by Astra-Zeneca, a pharmaceutical company that makes one of the proton-pump inhibitors. Astra-Zeneca can be contacted at 1-800-236-9933.

www.sts.org/doc/4119
  A web site designed to answer questions about GERD and maintained by the Society of Thoracic Surgeons (401 N. Michigan Ave., Chicago, IL 60611-4267; 312-644-6610).

www.sages.org/sg—pub22.html

"SAGES Guidelines for Surgical Treatment of Gastroesophageal Reflux Disease." A web site maintained by the Society of American Gastrointestinal Endoscopic Surgeons (2716 Ocean Park Blvd., Suite 3000, Santa Monica, CA 90405).

www.gastro.com/heartbrn.htm

An impartial and informative web site maintained by the National Digestive Diseases Information Clearing House (2 Information Way, Bethesda, MD 20892-3570).

www.mayo.edu.healthinfo

A web site maintained by the Mayo Clinic. The site is devoted primarily to the discussion of medications used for acid reflux.

www.jeffersonhealth.org.diseases.digestive-disorders/hrtburn.htm

A web site providing information on the causes and treatment of GERD maintained by the Jefferson Health System in Philadelphia.

www.allhealth.com/heartburn

A web site that answers questions about heartburn, and a chat room for discussions among people with heartburn.

www.healthanswers.com

A web site designed to answer basic questions about all types of health issues.

www.healthylives.com

A web site maintained by Glaxo-Wellcome, a pharmaceutical company, to answer questions about heartburn.

galen.med.virginia.edu

A web site maintained by the Medical College of Virginia that focuses on children's health issues. A good site for basic information concerning acid reflux disease in children.

www.niddk.nih.gov/health/digest/digest.htm

A web site maintained by United States National Institutes of Health that can be used to access information on all types of digestive disorders and gastrointestinal diseases.

Index

acetaminophen, 79
acid reflux. *See* gastroesophageal reflux disease (GERD)
Aciphex. *See* rabeprazole
adenocarcinoma, 133
air trapping, 41
alcohol, 76, 96, 127
alginic acid (Gaviscon), 84–85, 143,
158–59
Alka-Seltzer, 86
AlternaGEL, 86–87
aluminum, 82
aluminum hydroxide, 85, 86–87, 88
aluminum sucrose sulfate, 85
amnesia, 63
Amphojel, 87
anemia, iron-deficiency, 127
anesthetics, as used during upper endoscopy, 53–54, 62–65
angina pectoris, 34
antacids, 5–6, 7, 85–90; cautions regarding, 82; for children, 138; during pregnancy, 143; and tetracycline, 84, 87, 88, 89, 90
antihistamines, 65
antibiotics. *See* clarithromycin;
erythromycin; tetracycline
anxiolytics, 63

argon plasma coagulation (APC),
168–69
ascertainment bias, 119
ascites, 31
aspiration pneumonia, 36
aspirin, 79
asthma and GERD, 30, 37–41, 98,
139
Axid / Axid AR. *See* nizatidine

bad breath, 44
baking soda, 92–93
barium sulfate, 51
barium swallow (esophagram), 23,
50–52, 58, 105, 124, 141
Barrett's esophagus, 6, 8, 18, 56, 57,
58, 96–97, 124, 128–29, 148; blood
test for, 164–65; diagnosis of, 164–
67; treatment of, 130–31, 167–69
bed-bound patients, 149–50
belching, 31
Benadryl, 65
benzocaine, 53, 64
bile, 18–19
biopsies, 8, 54, 56, 124–25. *See also*
cancer, esophageal
bite block, 54
bleeding, esophageal, 126–28

bone weakening (osteomalacia), 82, 87
bougienage, 125
bread, 93
breastfeeding and medications, 81, 90, 91, 92, 145
bronchoconstriction, 37
bronchodilators, 40
bronchospasm, 37, 39
buttermilk, 93

calcium, 82
calcium carbonate, 87, 89–90
calcium-channel blockers, 61, 79, 147
calcium glycerophosphate, 89
cancer, esophageal, 131–34; and Barrett's esophagus, 128–29, 130; treatment for, 133–34
Candida albicans, 120
Carafate, 85
carcinoma of the esophagus. *See* cancer, esophageal
Cetacaine, 64
chest pain, 34–36, 48, 98
children, GERD and, 135–39
cimetidine (Tagamet), 39, 90, 92, 99, 100, 145–46
cisapride (Propulsid), 103–4, 157
citrus products, 20
clarithromycin, 103
cola drinks, 71
colon, 12
colonoscopy, 127
columnar epithelium, 17
columnar mucosa, 17, 21
congenital hernia, 22
conscious sedation, 53, 62–63, 141
constipation, 82, 86, 90
cough, chronic, 41–44, 48, 137
Coumadin. *See* warfarin
CT scans, 162

Demerol, 64
dental erosions, 44
Depo-Provera, 155–56
diarrhea, 82
diazepam (Valium), 63, 64
differential diagnosis, 49
diffuse esophageal spasm, 35–36
Di-Gel, 82, 87
digestive system, 11–13
dilation. *See* esophageal dilation
diltiazem, 61
drugs. *See* over-the-counter medicines; prescription medicines
duodenum, 8
dysphagia. *See* swallowing difficulties

ear pain, 44
edema, 37
EGD. *See* esophagogastroduodenoscopy
elderly people and GERD, 29, 147–49
empiric treatment. *See* therapeutic trials
endoscope, 54, 161–62
endoscopic suturing, 111, 159–60
endoscopist, 50
endoscopy. *See* colonoscopy; esophagogastroduodenoscopy
enzyme precursor, 14
erosion, esophageal, 58, 119
erythromycin, 103
esomeprazole (Nexium), 39, 43, 102, 121, 147. *See also* proton-pump inhibitors
esophageal dilation, 125–26
esophageal hiatus, 13, 20. *See also* hiatal hernia
esophageal manometry, 60–62, 110, 141, 162
esophageal motility disorders, 35–36, 60–62, 107, 147–48

esophageal mucosa, 17, 52, 57–58

esophageal rings, 122–23

esophageal sphincter. *See* lower esophageal sphincter; upper esophageal sphincter

esophageal varices, 126–27

esophagitis, 8, 23, 27, 28, 29, 33, 57, 96, 106, 118–20; and chronic bleeding, 127–28; erosive, 126; treatment of, 120–21

esophagogastroduodenoscopy (EGD, or upper endoscopy), 7–8, 23, 49, 53–58, 96, 101, 105, 110, 124, 168; for diagnosis of Barrett's esophagus, 165–66; improvements in, 161–62; limitations of, 56–57; medications used during, 62–65; during pregnancy, 50, 141–42

esophagram. *See* barium swallow

esophagus, 8, 13–14; bleeding in, 126–28; defense mechanisms of, 16–17

Extra Strength Maalox, 87–88, 94

famotidine (Pepcid), 39, 90, 91–92, 99

fat, dietary, as factor in GERD, 75–76

fentanyl, 64

fistula, 136

flumazenil, 63

food impaction, 123

fundoplication. *See* Nissen fundoplication

gas bloat syndrome, 110

gastric secretions, 14

gastroenterologist, 7

gastroesophageal junction, 15, 16–18, 21, 160

gastroesophageal reflux disease (GERD), 6; age as factor in, 29, 147–49; antacids as treatment for, 5–6; and asthma, 30, 37–41; asymptomatic, 27–28; and Barrett's esophagus, 128–31; and bed-bound patients, 149–50; and bleeding, 126–28; and cancer, 131–34; chest pain as symptom of, 34–36; in children, 135–39; chronic cough as symptom of, 41–44; complications of, 115–34, 164–69; diagnosis of, 47–65, 161–64; in elderly people, 29, 147–49; and esophagitis, 118–21; future of treatment for, 154–59; head and neck symptoms of, 44–46; heartburn as symptom of, 30–31; and hiatal hernia, 23; lifestyle modifications as response to, 69–79; lung symptoms of, 36–44; misconceptions about, 18–20; obesity as risk factor, 76–77; and pregnancy, 9, 49–50, 76–77, 139–47; prevention of, 70; regurgitation as symptom of, 31–32, 47–48; risk factors for, 9–10, 76–78; seeking medical attention for, 97–98; and smoking, 77–78; and strictures, 121–26; surgery for, 105–11, 130, 159–61; and swallowing difficulties, 33–34; symptoms of, 4–5, 6, 9, 16–17, 27–46, 97–98, 116–18, 149–50; tests for, 49–65, 98, 161–64; treatment of, 5–6, 9, 98–99; water brash as symptom of, 32–33, 48, 149. *See also* over-the-counter medicines; prescription medicines

gastrograffin, 51

gastrointestinal tract, 12–13

gastrum, 8

Gaviscon. *See* alginic acid

GE junction. *See* gastroesophageal junction

Gelusil, 82, 87
generic medicines, 99
glucagon, 65

heart attack, 34–35
heartburn: as symptom of GERD, 18, 30–31, 47, 139–40; as symptom of esophagitis, 119. *See also* gastro-esophageal reflux disease (GERD)
heart failure and over-the-counter medication, 82
hernia. *See* hiatal hernia
hiatal hernia, 8, 13, 20, 21, 22, 23, 148
hiatus, 13
histamine type 2 blockers. *See* H_2-blockers
hoarseness, 44, 45, 48, 98, 137
H_2-blockers, 5, 39–40, 44, 104, 121, 156; for bed-bound patients, 150; for children, 138; doses, 90–92, 99; over-the-counter, 90–92, 94; during pregnancy, 143, 145; prescription, 99–101, 104; side effects, 100
Hurricane spray, 64
hydrochloric acid, 14
hydroxyzine (Vistaril), 65

ibuprofen, 79
ice cream, 93
indirect laryngoscopy, 45
infants. *See* children, GERD and
intestinal metaplasia, 133
intestines. *See* colon; small intestine
iron-deficiency anemia, 127
iron supplements, 120

ketoconazole, 100, 103
kidney function, 82, 86, 87–88, 89
kidney stones, 82, 90

lansoprazole (Prevacid), 32, 33, 39, 43, 96, 102, 103, 104, 121, 138, 147. *See also* proton-pump inhibitors
laparoscopic Nissen fundoplication. *See* Nissen fundoplication
laryngitis, 44, 45
larynx, 44–45
LES. *See* lower esophageal sphincter
lidocaine spray, 64
lifestyle modifications, 69–73; for bed-bound patients, 150; body position, 73–75; eating habits, 71–73, 75–76; medicines, 78–79; during pregnancy, 142; smoking, 77–78; tight clothing, 78
liquid nitrogen, 167
lower esophageal sphincter (LES), 15, 16, 157–58, 162; foods and medicines that affect, 19, 31, 75–77, 78–79; during pregnancy, 140; surgery for, 106–7, 108–11, 159–60

Maalox, 82–84, 87–88, 94, 143
magaldrate, 89
magnesium, 82
magnesium hydroxide, 87–90
magnesium trisilicate, 85
medications. *See* over-the-counter medicines; prescription medicines
meperidine (Demerol), 64
metoclopramide (Reglan), 61, 103–4, 106, 138, 148, 158
microaspiration, 37
midazolam (Versed), 63–64
milk, 93
Milk of Magnesia, Phillips', 88–89
morphine, 64
motility. *See* esophageal motility disorders

MRI (magnetic resonance imaging), 162

Mylanta, 88, 94, 105, 143

Mylanta AR Acid Reducer, 91, 92

Mylanta DS, 82, 88, 94

Mylanta II, 82

myocardial infarction. *See* heart attack

narcotics, 64

nefazodone (Serzone), 103

Nephrox suspension, 82, 88

Nexium. *See* esomeprazole

nicotine, 77–78

nifedipine, 61

Nissen fundoplication, 107, 108–11, 139, 159

nitrates, 61, 78, 147

nizatidine (Axid), 39, 90, 91, 99, 146–47

nonspecific esophageal motility disorder, 36

nutcracker esophagus, 35

obesity, as factor in GERD, 76–77

occult blood, 127

omeprazole (Prilosec), 7, 39, 43, 99, 102–3, 104–6, 121, 138, 147. *See also* proton-pump inhibitors

opioids, 64

osteomalacia. *See* bone weakening

over-the-counter medicines, 80–84; antacids, 85–90; cautions regarding, 94–95; home remedies, 92–93; H_2–blockers, 90–92; improvements in, 156; and pregnancy, 81–82, 90, 91, 92; recommendations, 93–95; side effects, 82, 90–91; topical agents, 84–85

palliative treatments, 133–34

pancreatic juices, 19

pantoprazole (Protonix), 39, 43, 102, 103, 121, 155. *See also* proton-pump inhibitors

paraesophageal hernia, 21–22, 23–24

partial wrap, 110–11

Pepcid AC Acid Controller, 91–92. *See also* famotidine

pepsin, 14, 19–20, 85–86

pepsinogen, 14, 19

peptic strictures. *See* strictures

perforation, 56, 109

peristalsis, 13

pharynx, 13, 44, 45

Phenergan, 65

phenytoin, 92, 100

Phillips' Milk of Magnesia, 88–89

photodynamic therapy (PDT), 168

pH probe. *See* 24–hour pH probe

physiologic reflux, 16, 115

pneumonia, 36, 137

polyps, vocal cord, 44, 45

postnasal drip, 44

potassium, 120, 122

pregnancy: and GERD, 9, 49–50, 76–77, 139–47; lifestyle modifications during, 142; medications during, 81–82, 90, 91, 92, 142, 143–47; tests during, 141–42

Prelief, 89

prescribing doctor, 50

prescription medicines, 96–99; H_2–blockers, 99–101, 104; improvements in, 154–59; prokinetic agents, 103–4, 157–58; proton-pump inhibitors, 101–3, 104–5

Prevacid. *See* lansoprazole

Prilosec. *See* omeprazole

projectile vomiting, 136

prokinetic agents, 103–4, 106, 138, 148, 157–58, 163

promethazine, 65
Propofol, 65
Propulsid (cisapride), 103–4
prostate-specific antigen (PSA) test, 164
proton-pump inhibitors, 7, 8, 32, 33, 39–40, 96, 97, 101–3, 104–6, 107–8, 111, 148, 154–55, 156, 163; for Barrett's esophagus, 130; for bed-bound patients, 150; for children, 138; doses, 101–2, 104–5; for chronic cough, 43–44; for esophagitis, 121, 127–28; during pregnancy, 147; side effects, 102
Protonix. See pantoprazole
pulmonary fibrosis, 36
pyloric stenosis, 136
pylorus, 14, 54, 136
pyrosis. See heartburn

rabeprazole (Aciphex), 39, 43, 102, 121, 147. See also proton-pump inhibitors
radiologist, 50
radio-opaque liquids, 50–51
ranitidine (Zantac), 6–7, 39, 90, 92, 99, 117, 145
reflex mechanism, 37, 39
reflux mechanism, 37
Reglan. See metoclopramide
regurgitation: during pregnancy, 140; as symptom of GERD, 18, 31–32, 47–48; as symptom of GERD in children, 136; as symptom of esophagitis, 119
renal insufficiency. See kidney function
reporting bias, 73
Retrovir, 103
Riopan, 89
Rolaids, 82, 89–90, 94

saliva, 31–32. See also water brash
salt-restricted diets, 82
Schatzki's B rings, 122–23
sedatives, 63–64
Serzone (nefazodone), 103
simethicone, 87, 88, 94
sleep apnea, 36
sliding hernia, 21
small intestine, 13
smoking, as factor in GERD, 77–78
sodium, 82
sodium bicarbonate, 86, 92–93
sore throat, 44
sphincter, 16
spicy foods, 20
squamous cell carcinoma, 133
squamous epithelium, 17, 164–65
squamous mucosa, 17, 21
stents, 134
stomach, 13, 14
stomach hernias, 21–24. See also hiatal hernia; paraesophageal hernia
stools, blood in, 126
strangulated hernia, 24
Stretta procedure, 111, 160–61
strictures, 27–28, 33–34, 117–18, 121–26, 128
Sublimaze, 64
sucralfate, 85
sudden infant death syndrome (SIDS), 137
surgery, 105–11, 130; future of, 159–61
swallowing difficulties, 33–34, 97, 110, 117–18, 121–22, 137
symptomatic treatment, 101
symptoms of GERD, 4–5, 6, 9, 16–17, 27–30, 97–98, 116–18; asthma, 30, 37–41, 98, 139; in bed-bound patients, 149–50; chest pain, 34–36, 48, 98; in children, 136–37;

chronic cough, 41–44, 48, 137; in the elderly, 147–48; in the head and neck, 44–46; heartburn, 18, 30–31, 47, 139–40; in pregnant women, 140–41; regurgitation, 18, 31–32, 47–48, 136; swallowing difficulties, 33–34, 97, 110, 117–18, 121–22, 137; water brash, 32–33, 48, 140, 149

Tagamet. *See* cimetidine
Tagamet HB 200, 92, 96. *See also* cimetidine
technician, 50
tests, diagnostic. *See* barium swallow; esophageal manometry; esophagogastroduodenoscopy; 24–hour pH probe; upper gastrointestinal series
tetracycline, 84, 87, 88, 89, 90, 120
theophylline, 40–41, 61, 78–79, 92, 100, 147
therapeutic trials, 32, 48, 141
thermal injury, 160
throat problems, 44
tight clothing, 78
tinnitus, 86
Titralac, 82, 90
Titralac Extra Strength, 90
tomato products, 20
topical agents, 84–85

topical anesthetics, 53, 64–65
Tums, 90, 94
24–hour pH probe, 8, 32–33, 43, 45, 58–60, 107, 110, 141, 162–63

ulcer, esophageal, 58, 119
upper endoscopy. *See* esophagogastroduodenoscopy
upper esophageal sphincter, 16
upper gastrointestinal series, 23, 52–53, 141

Valium (diazepam), 63, 64
verapamil, 61
Versed. *See* midazolam
Vistaril. *See* hydroxyzine
vocal cord polyps, 44, 45
vomiting, 97. *See also* regurgitation

warfarin (Coumadin), 92, 100, 102
water brash, 32–33, 48, 140, 149
wheezing, 37, 39, 137, 149. *See also* asthma

x-rays. *See* barium swallow; esophagogastroduodenoscopy; upper gastrointestinal series
Xylocaine, 64

Zantac. *See* ranitidine
Zantac 75, 92. *See also* ranitidine